WATER EXERCISES

WATER

EXERCISES

ANTHONY HARRIS

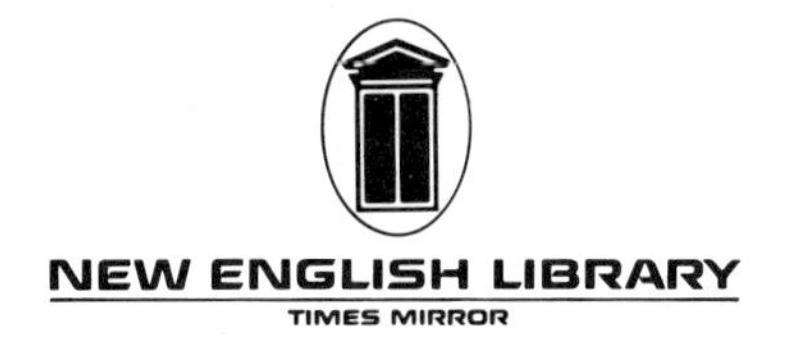

NEW ENGLISH LIBRARY
TIMES MIRROR

Editor: Nicola Davies
Art Editor: Deborah Miles
Design: Michael Osborn
Illustrations: Joyce Smith and David Dowland

This edition published in 1979 by
New English Library Limited,
Barnard's Inn, Holborn, London EC1N 2JR, England

Text Filmset in Palatino by Modern Text Typesetting,
2 Carlton Court, Grainger Road, Southend-on-Sea, Essex.

Printed in Great Britain by M. and A. Thomson Litho,
East Kilbride, Scotland.
Bound by Hunter and Foulis, Edinburgh, Scotland.

CONTENTS

WATER EXERCISES

INTRODUCTION

This book tells you in a simple, sound way, how to use the sea, swimming-pool, bath or shower to gain a healthier, more shapely body. The exercises are unique, enjoyable and good to look at, and break entirely new ground in figure maintenance, reduction of stress, and the building up of stamina with vitality for your everyday work and play.

Water is an ideal medium in which to exercise because it makes the body virtually weightless, allowing you to use specific movements for specific points of your body in a new and concentrated way. It also provides resistance for your body to work against, and both stimulates the skin and relaxes the muscles. Water is also a cleansing element, soothing, yet taking away sweat and dead skin from your body, and it creates a superb surface for massage.

The exercises in this book can be done easily in the sea, in a swimming-pool, or indeed in any body of water. Generally, they have been adapted for use when the current is low. Most exercises, too, can be done entirely alone, but often a partner can be used, in place of the side support along the edge of a swimming-pool. Each exercise is graded for specific body-area shaping. Such is the versatility of the water exercise that if you want to use the exercises to slim, you perform them more quickly, but with the minimum of resistance in the water, which means that you use a minimum depth for your body. If you want to build tissue and strength you must move as hard as you can in the greatest depth of water so that you have more water resistance. Men who wish to build a strong body can utilise this principle, but women will find that they can develop superbly shaped and strong bodies, without any evidence of excessive bulging muscles at all by using the standard exercises in the depth of water recommended.

As the body becomes stronger, so the heart will also become stronger, which is essential to an active, healthy life. If you are unfit your heart will react wildly to exertion and beat far more than is necessary. Even when you stop, it will continue to beat in this exaggerated manner, only coming to its resting phase long after. This means that your heart is working much harder for longer periods than the exertion demands. The exercises in this book are designed specially to be a gradual and gentle improvement programme for you to do at your own pace, without strain. The general principle is that if an exercise feels bad and you have to make a huge effort, it is doing you no good at all. The exercises here are based on pleasure and should be fun and stimulating to try, and once you get fit you can stay fit with just a few minutes every day.

Water Exercises is devoted to emphasising natural power, your natural vitality and beauty and your natural pleasure in feeling fitter, and more aware of your body. All the exercises and techniques share these features:

- ☐ they are enjoyable
- ☐ they increase the strength of the heart
- ☐ they remove excess fat
- ☐ they improve your capacity to relax
- ☐ they arrest the process of ageing by deterioration
- ☐ they more rapidly remove waste products from your blood.
- ☐ they are good to look at
- ☐ they shape the body
- ☐ they increase vitality and endurance for daily living
- ☐ they increase the flow of blood to and from your tissues

By following the schedules in this book, you can achieve and maintain an excellent natural fitness that will make you feel stronger, slimmer, invigorated and relaxed.

FACTS TO WORK

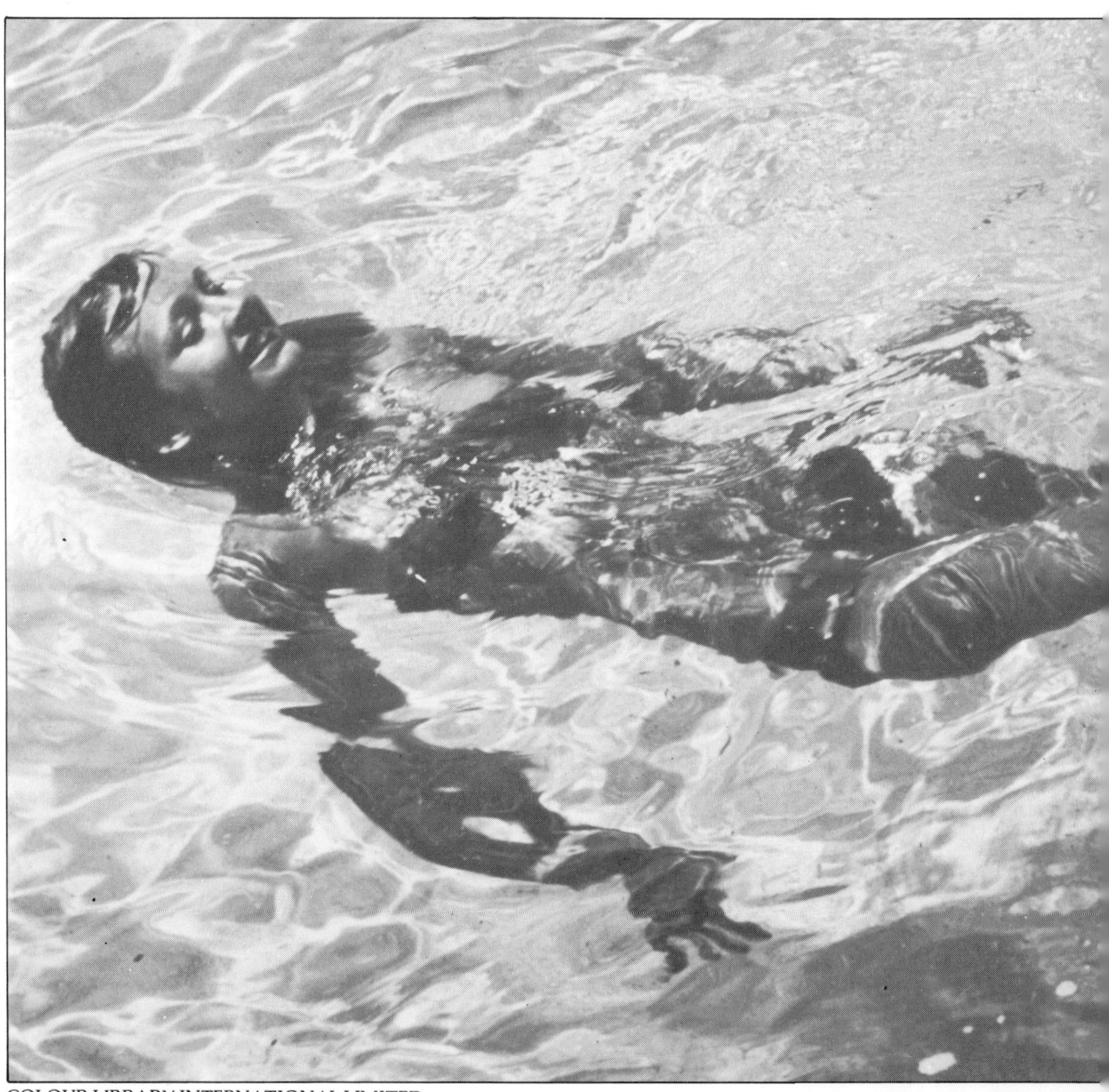

COLOUR LIBRARY INTERNATIONAL LIMITED

WITH

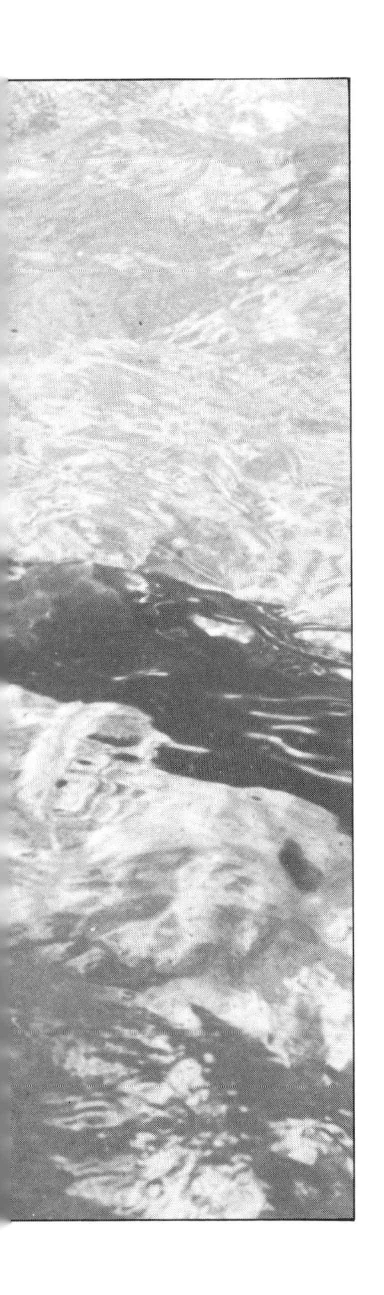

1 When you are being supported by water you are virtually weightless, thus your muscles can work against water resistance.

2 The force you exert can be up to five times more than when running. Therefore, you use more muscles when swimming, with greater efficiency.

3 You need to balance your energy intake by eating well as explained.

4 Women's work-rates are less than men's but this difference nearly vanishes when we make allowances for their smaller size and less muscle, pound for pound of body, than men. This means water exercises can be adapted to suit women and men equally well.

5 Because you are weightless in the water, the exercises can be concentrated on specific points of your body for figure, health and firmness.

6 Water exercises are suitable for people who are very unfit because they can be performed with minimal exertion or strain, yet, because the exercises can be adapted to greater depths, with increased effort, they can be used for maximum effect too.

Chapter One

FITNESS AND SHAPE

FITNESS AND SHAPE

Excellent natural fitness can be easily achieved and maintained without too much trouble by working through the schedules of this book. It is important to start gently and allow your body to adapt. Gradually you can work up to the higher levels, but in any case the amount of time required is minutes rather than hours. This chapter is devoted to emphasising natural power, your natural beauty and your natural pleasure in your own body, and gives you detailed tables for the kind of weight/shape you should have, and the type of exercises with which you should begin.

Fitness

Endurance, which in effect is another way of speaking about fitness, is built up by gradually increasing your exercise load. There is, however, no point in getting yourself to the super-fitness level of Olympic athletes, for example, because all this means is that you will have to spend many hours every day to reach, then maintain, that level. When you stop, your level of fitness will fall rapidly.

If we call excellent fitness 100 units, then super-fitness is, say, 120 units, while average fitness is about 30. It takes only a little effort, but one that must be sustained over several weeks or months depending on your general health, to reach excellent fitness, and only a small attention several minutes a day, as long as you eat well, to keep at 100 units; but each point after that is very hard won indeed.

I believe that the fitness levels of international athletes are freakish and do not represent any special merit as far as shape and beauty are concerned, being hot-house examples of unnatural over-development and excessive dedication. The level of fitness aimed for in this book, however, is that of a perfectly functioning body well able to meet life's challenge.

The fact is that most people live far below this level. The longer you live below it, the shorter your life, and the less physically attractive you are. It will also take you much longer to reach this level of fitness. On the other hand, the 100 units at forty years of age is only a little different from the 100 units at twenty. This means that an excellently fit fifty-year-old is in better shape than, and can out-compete, an out-of-condition twenty-five-year-old. Indeed, the more research we do on this subject, the more we realise that what we think of as the inevitable deterioration in the body as being age is not age at all, but neglect and deterioration caused by stress, poor food and lack of exercise.

STRESS

Stress is when a natural function of your body has been tried and tested beyond its capacity to stand up to the strain imposed upon it. This can occur through repeated small strains, as for instance not sweating, not exercising, not eating well, or by some big strain like being hit by a car, or a sudden blast of high-energy sound, or a drug. But the main cause of stress in our civilisation is tenseness caused by trying to meet deadlines, or through ignoring danger signals that come from your body.

If you try to feel what your body is doing, you will find out if you are stressed. If pain comes when you turn on to your body, don't be frightened. It means at last you are actually getting to know the real situation.

Stressed people cannot feel pleasure well. Another way of putting this is to say that if you are properly fit, you will feel pleasure every day.

I have graded the exercises in this book to reawaken your awareness of your own body. In time, as you learn to relax and use the exercise and massage movements, you will enjoy the increasingly pleasurable feelings of having a controlled and responsive body.

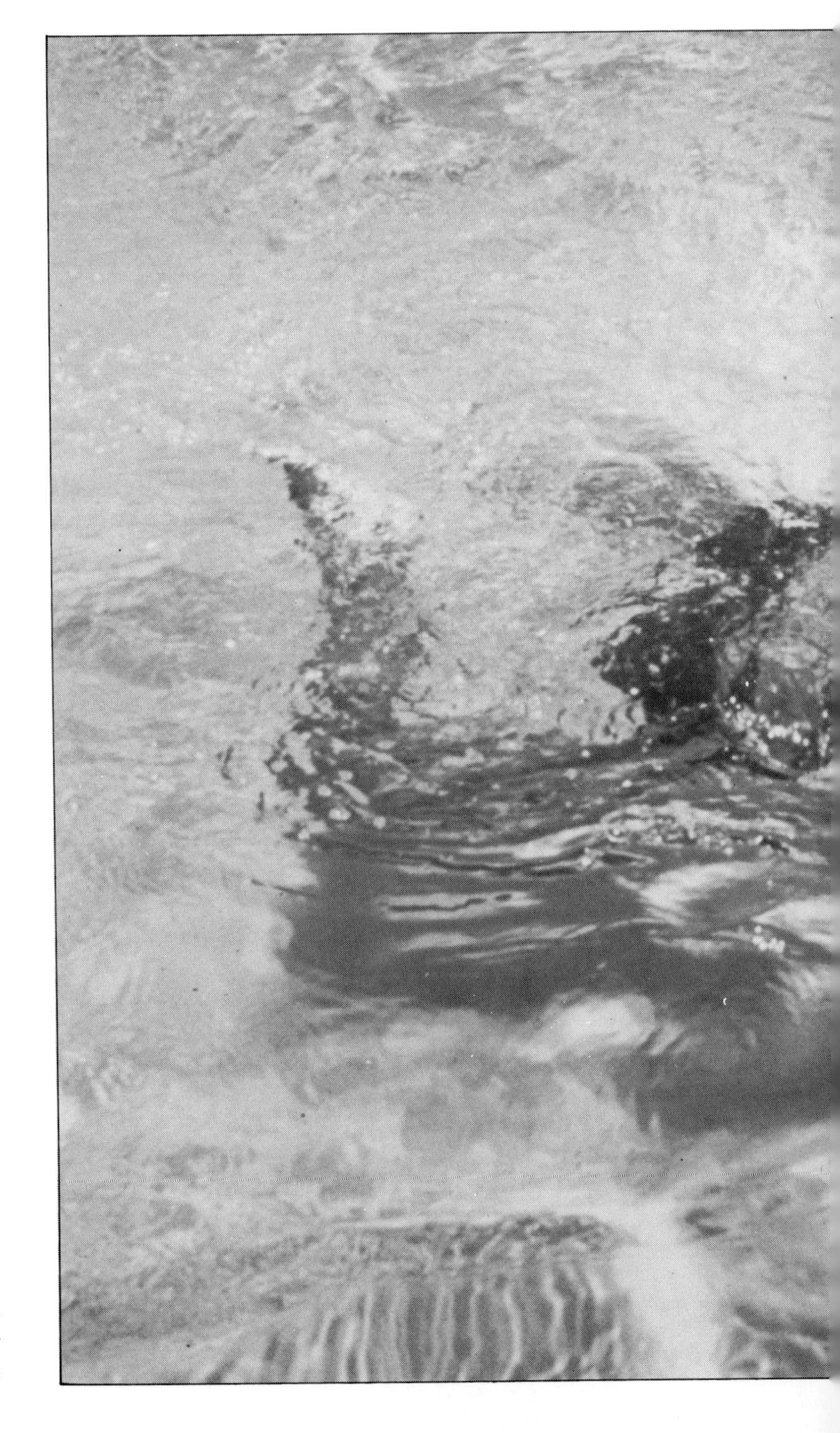

SWEATING

One of the advantages of working in water is that you don't ever feel unpleasantly overheated (unless the water is too hot!) because the sweat is being washed away.

We sweat constantly; even when we think we are not, we are losing water all over the body, particularly in the regions of the face, the armpits and the insides of the thighs. This sweating process enables us to lose heat, and so keep our blood and tissues at the right temperature for natural chemical reactions to proceed at the right speed. When we are too cold, our chemical reactions slow down—a condition of hypothermia—while if we are too hot, it is the condition we call fever. Both these conditions occur when the chemical reactions are disturbed by temperature. The other function of sweating is to get rid of waste

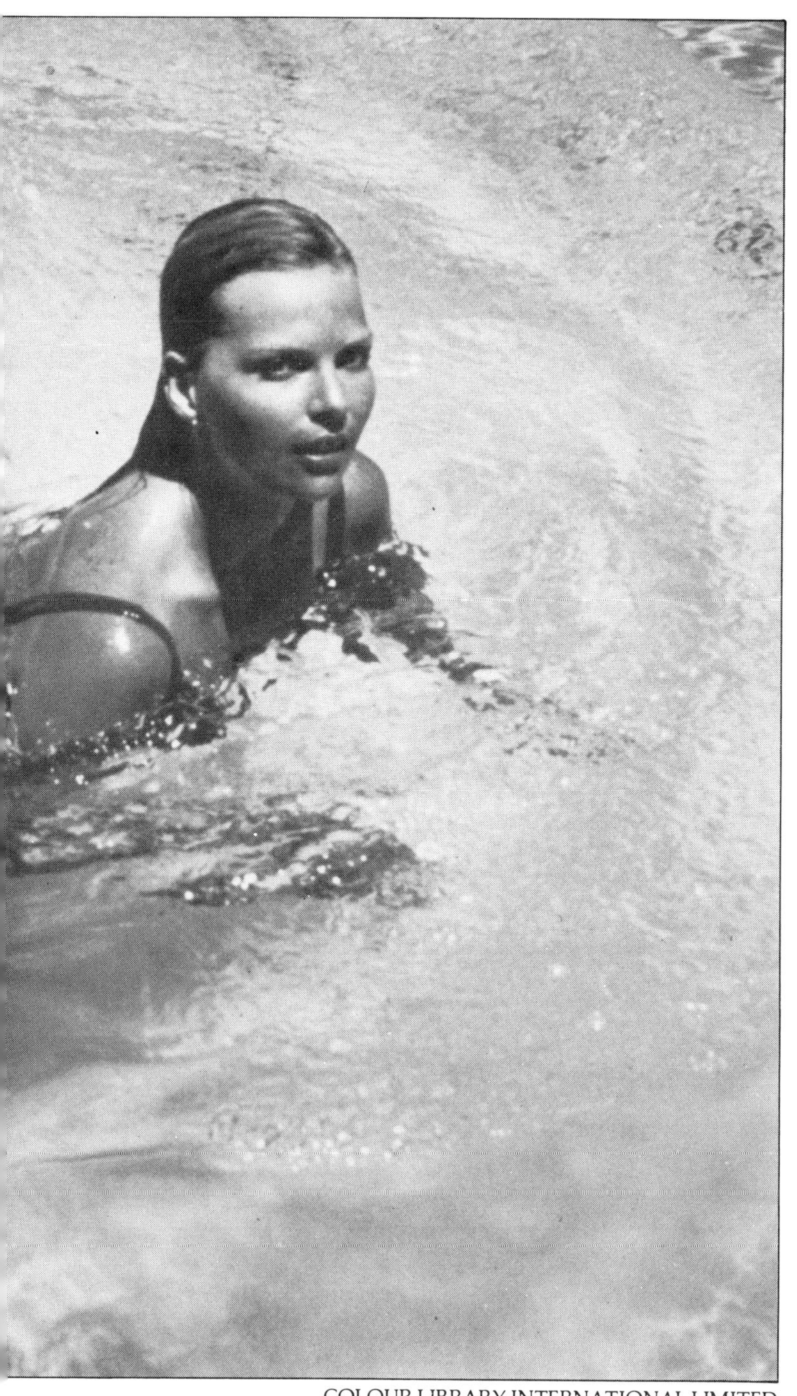
COLOUR LIBRARY INTERNATIONAL LIMITED

products, mostly urea and some salt, which must be kept low in the body. Indeed, when urea rises too high in the blood stream, it can be fatal.

At night we lose between a pint and two-and-a-half pints of fluid. You can see, then, that not to sweat is very unhealthy. Dogs cannot sweat through their skins, so they have long tongues and you'll have noticed how a dog hangs out his tongue on a hot day. If you put a deodorant over his tongue, a drying one, you would have a very sick dog in a short time. It might be an idea to remember this when next you spray yourself with a drying deodorant that stops your body working properly. Many of the headaches, general fatigue and bad breath found in city workers are caused by excessive use of drying deodorants.

THE HEART

A strong heart will still be beating easily even after the strongest muscles in the body have given up, totally tired out. It can peak 200 beats a minute in supreme effort and recover, to fall to 50, in perfect rest.

If you are fit your resting heart rate would be about 65-70 a minute. On exerting yourself it will climb to meet the demand for fresh blood in the muscles, but when you stop working it will fall very rapidly to its resting value. If you are unfit, your heart will react wildly to exertion, climbing 10, 20, 30, 60, even 100, beats *more* than is necessary for the exertion. Even when you stop, it will continue to beat in this exaggerated manner, only coming to its resting phase long after. This means that when you are unfit, your heart works much harder for longer periods than the exertion demands.

If you are overweight your heart has to work too hard for all that useless fat that you are carrying around. Change your eating habits by following the advice given later in this book.

When you go into a water exercise remember to do it gently at first, then gradually build up to more strenuous routines. Once you become fit it will require only a little time and effort to maintain that fitness.

Shape

Physical work-outs might make you fit but they can also make you ugly by developing your body in a poor way. If you go in for body weight, you can achieve it easily, but once you stop the three-hours-a-day grunting and sucking vitamin goo, you'll lose it all again. My experience convinces me that thin, bony men, say about 5 feet 10 inches, weighing 10 stones, should not embark on body-building exercises as such, but instead should toughen up their usually powerful and wiry bodies.

Very skinny girls never seem to know what to do. The secret is to eat good food—and exercise. Soon, the skin gets sleeker and the body will acquire a thin layer of fat, which all women should have, over the bones. Don't exercise, and the body will become gaunt: exercise and it will look great.

Big-boned men and women naturally tend to get fatter and fatter. Don't. Just eat wisely as explained in Chapter Two and get good lines and fitness by exercising in water.

This question of body image is so important. You cannot change your bone type—and why should you? Big men are attractive to women, and so are large girls to men: but big in bone, in frame, not big in fat. To make my point—and this might surprise you—a man who weighs 14 stones at 5 feet 10 inches without excess fat is a very big man, but there are few of them around although there are millions of men of 5 feet 10 inches who weigh 14 stone.

So, we have an inflated idea of what big is, because we go by overweight people in Europe and America. With women we have the opposite problem. So many thin girls are picked as models that normal-sized girls think they are too fat. If you cannot pinch more than half an inch anywhere you are not. What you probably are is slack in thighs, tummy and buttocks. Your muscles probably need tightening. You need to exercise.

One of the most beautiful women I have ever known was 5 feet 8 inches tall and weighed 10 stone 5 pounds, without the slightest trace of cellulite or excess fat. She was not butch. She seemed to be a sister of Michelangelo's 'Night' sculpture. And yet she wanted to weigh 9 stones. To do this, she would have ruined her health, her figure and her looks, and run the risk of destroying an outgoing vivacious personality.

Her trouble was that she didn't know who she was. Her hair was thick and luxuriant, her health abundant. She was a muscular woman. Once I made her understand that no matter what she did, this would always be true, her attitude towards herself changed; because she learned to capitalise on herself.

Even before you speak, your body tells people who you are. If you neglect it, people will feel that you will neglect them. If you respect and care for it, other people will feel that you will care for and respect them. Why not have a body which says what you want to say?

Jennifer was 5 feet 5 inches and weighed a petite and perfect 7 stone 10 pounds. She had blue eyes, fair hair, and was in excellent health. She loved fashionable clothes. Her expensive toilet, hair-style and cosmetics made her look like a gorgeous blonde doll—a doll, not a woman. Jennifer didn't really believe she had a body, she thought it was an accessory.

She complained of feeling artificial, empty. This attractive twenty-two-year-old university student reading history, fell into the poor-little-rich-girl syndrome.

Her parents made her go the rounds of psychologists who spoke of double-binds, but Jennifer became more remote, more and more unhappy, until she drifted into apathy. This was a curious apathy; she took on the reverse of her former over-dressed image, the blonde doll became a rag-doll. She dressed badly, got fat, hated her physical self, proclaimed that nothing much mattered. She fed her mind with books and her body with sweets. She exercised herself on the Corn Laws but let her body languish. She failed her degree.

Jennifer had never come to terms with her physical self, and her personality along with her academic career deteriorated the longer her ignorance persisted. She had to learn how to see that she was a physical person, a sweating, breathing organism. Not a doll, but a mature human person, a mature female body. Not a brain only, but glands and other organs too.

Whenever you do anything, you use your body. Einstein used his brain, a part of his body. The Queen honours occasions most when she is physically present. Margot Fonteyn uses her bones and muscles to entertain us in dance. Olivier's acting is a physical skill. Yehudi Menuhin uses fingers and skin to make his violin speak to us. Children know they are loved when they are touched. You cannot do anything without your body. So why not get the best out of it?

Everyone knows we should look after our bodies but the question remains—how?

Should you run up and down on the spot? Sue's ankles were bruised, thick and painful. She'd been following a course which told her to run on the spot. Thousands of people have done it, jarring themselves. She learned how to exercise properly to give herself shape and pleasure.

Should you jog through filthy city streets on hard pavements in cold weather? In Hampstead I see heavy-busted women jogging along furiously, almost certainly tearing the tissues of their breasts.

Should you starve yourself and become shrivelled in face, shapeless in body? Should you force yourself into exercise that is neither beneficial nor pleasurable? Or is there another way?

The exercises in this book will not turn a girl into an Amazon, but they will make her better-looking and happier with herself. For men, the need is to get rid of the flab and put on muscle. Often just two pounds only are required. With these water exercises there is no sweating with iron, no early-morning jogging. You can have fun *and* build up your natural fitness and power. They are designed to combine leanness with vigour, and to give fitness and shape. Indeed the two are inseparable in my philosophy. Beauty is fitness, fitness is beauty. Mere mechanical efficiency sells you short, not as short as unfitness but still short.

STRENGTH AND WEAKNESS IN SPORTS

Sport	Deficiency	Remedy
Running	Lack of arm and shoulder strength.	Crawl, breast-stroke, arm exercises.
Tennis	Assymetry of arm development, right over left.	Crawl, breast-stroke, arm exercises.
Boxing	Shortening of muscles. Lack of stretching.	Relaxation exercises, water massage.
Football	Lack of arm development.	Crawl, butterfly, arm exercises.
Karate	Hard, excessive rectilinear movement.	Shaping exercises.
Golf	Stress in back.	Back exercises.

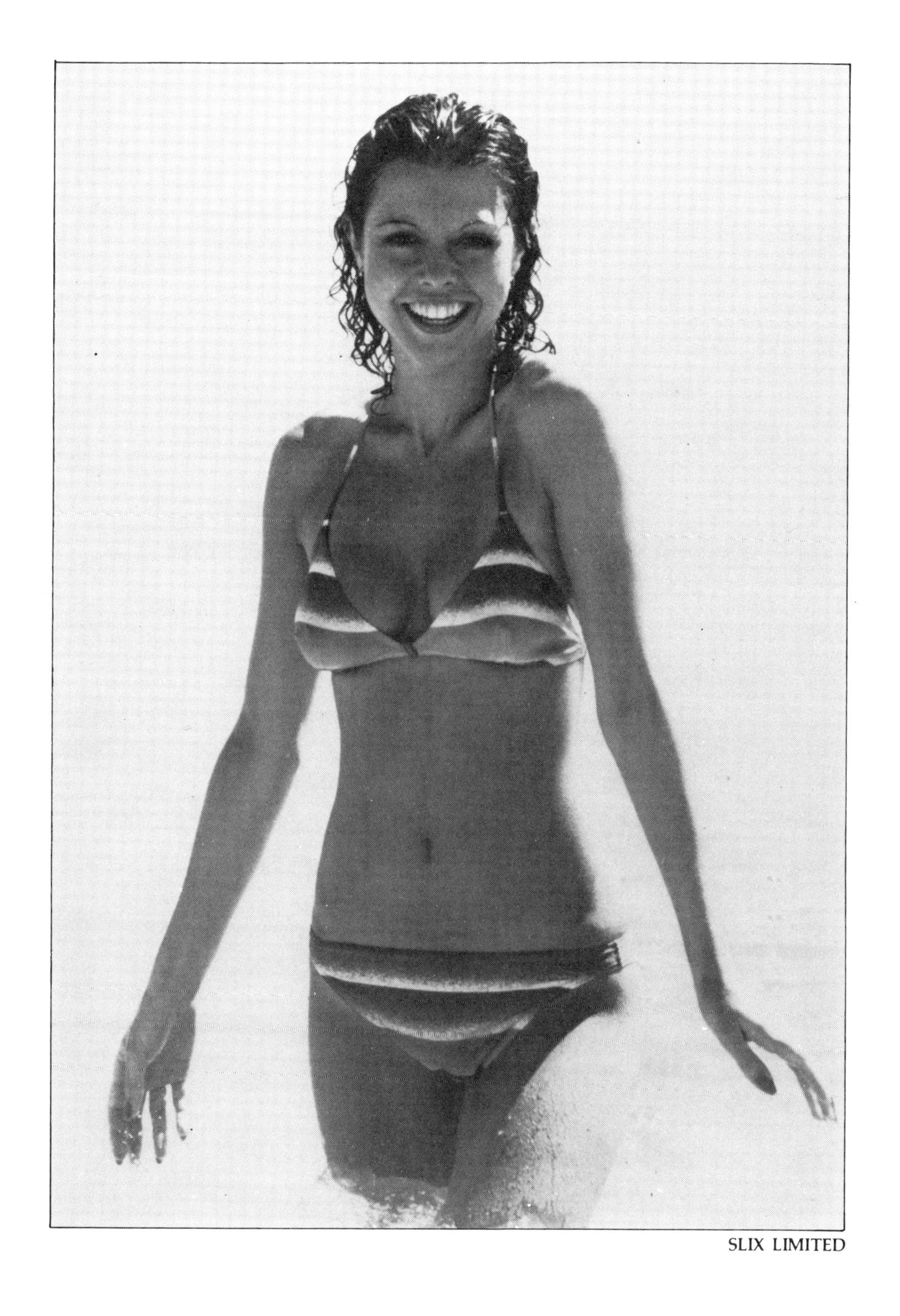

SLIX LIMITED

TABLE TWO: Weight in pounds for excellent figure shape for different skeletal types in men and women.

	←	Women	→	← Men		→
Frames Height	1	2	3	4	5	6
5ft	100	104	112	118	123	127
5ft 1in	103	107	115	121	126	130
5ft 2in	106	110	119	124	129	134
5ft 3in	109	113	123	127	133	138
5ft 4in	112	117	128	131	137	142
5ft 5in	116	121	132	135	141	146
5ft 6in	120	125	135	139	145	150
5ft 7in	124	129	139	144	149	155
5ft 8in	128	133	142	149	154	160
5ft 9in	132	137	146	154	159	165
5ft 10in	136	141	150	159	164	170
5ft 11in	140	145	155	164	169	176

These figure weights refer to men and women aged 25 years and in good health. The heights are without shoes, weights nude. If you are 18-24, move down one category, since it is perfectly normal to continue to grow tissue up to 25; thereafter growth tends to be extra weight.

How to use this chart
Frame One is very slight, ankles of less than 7 inches, wrists less than 6 inches. Women with this frame can still be very curved because the waistline accentuates the rest of the body. Men this small can enjoy swimming to move up to weight category Two. Frame Two is a medium frame. Men with this frame can move up to Frame Three weights with muscle, but in women, this usually means fat rather than muscle. The large frames Five and Six are generally for men with wrists of 7½ inches or more, and heavily muscled. There are seldom women of this size who have not an excess of fat.

IMPORTANT MUSCLES

Here is a list of figure-firming, fitness-essential muscles

Trapezius: the large muscle giving the curve of the shoulder from the back of the neck to the shoulder bone above the arm

Spinal erector muscles: these lie alongside the spinal column

Pectoral muscles: beneath the breasts

Abdominals: these lie in the centre of the abdomen reaching down from the rib-cage to the pubic area

Gluteals: the large muscles of the buttocks.

These muscles are particularly important to your strength, shape and fitness. The routines in this book will show you how to exercise them.

Chapter Two

ENERGY AND FOOD

ENERGY AND FOOD

Anyone who wishes to be slim, healthy and full of vitality and to remain so for the rest of his or her life, must learn to eat balanced, healthy and appetising food which will satisfy hunger, provide all the necessary vitamins, minerals, fats and proteins, and give pleasure. Healthy eating is essential for energy and warmth, the growth and repair of body tissues, and the protection and maintenance of our bodies.

Energy

You cannot work without using up energy. The amounts used can be measured very accurately. The average woman uses up 1,400 units of energy a day simply by being alive, but if she works as well, her over-all expenditure is about 2,300 calories. For the average man, the values are 1,700 and 3,000 calories a day.

Work rates are graded from light to excessive. For example, when sleeping you use up about 1 calorie a minute; in the office about 2 to 3 calories a minute. The grading of industrial work is as follows:

	Calories per minute	
	Men	**Women**
Light	3	2
Moderate	6	4
Heavy	8	6
Very Heavy	11	8
Excessive	12+	9+

Excessive industrial work is mining and lumber-working for example, while heavy work is hard manual labour. Other activities are shown below:

	Activities in calories per minute	
	Men	**Women**
Standing	3	2
Washing/driving	3.0	2.5
Sitting activities	1.5	1.0
Table-tennis, cricket	4	3
Hockey, tennis	6	5
Boxing	7.5	—
Squash	7.5	6.0
Laboratory work	2	1.8
Cooking	3.5	3
Hanging out washing	3.5	3
Bedmaking	4	3.5
Shopping with heavy load	5	4
Typing (40 wpm) mechanical	2	2
Typing (40 wpm) electric	2	2
Office work (sitting)	1	1
Sleeping	1	1

During sports activity your work rate sometimes rises above excessive work levels, but the average always falls below this over a period. In industrial work the expenditure is more even, and that is why above 9 to 10 for men and 8 for women is excessive; but in sport, short bursts of activity at this level are part of the beneficial effects of exercise.

Cross-country running means an expenditure of about 11 calories per minute, while average values for young people in shorter running distances range from 5 to 18 for men, 8 to 13 for women per minute; the upper levels are for hard, driving, running, usually with some sprinting or change of pace. A brisk walk consumes about 5 calories per minute on the level, more on a gradient. Swimming produces expenditures of between 5 and 18, the higher level for hard underwater swimming, or sprinting, the lower level for a brisk work out. If you swim in a very relaxed fashion you could be using only 2 or 3 calories a minute, while if you float in warmish water the expenditure is as if you were asleep.

Food and Diet

When you balance food intake with activity you will stay at the same weight, but if you overeat, you will put on extra poundage. You must first make sure that you are eating correctly, and then you can go on to build your figure properly by working through the courses in the text. When you are your correct weight you must work to keep and improve your figure, because you could be the right weight and still have it in the wrong places.

A woman radiates about 1,400 calories, and a man 1,700 calories a day, in a temperate climate; more in cold weather, less in hot. This is the basic loss of heat from the skin. Since an average woman eats the equivalent of 2,300 calories a day, and a man 3,000, in sedentary jobs there is a leeway of 900 for a woman, 1,300 for a man. A pound of fatty tissue has the energy equivalent of about 3,500 calories, and, therefore, if you sit around doing little, in a short time you will become very fat indeed. For instance, if you had a surfeit of 900 calories a day, in four days you would put on one pound in fat, or about half a stone in a month. By the end of the year you would be grossly overweight.

Fat is twice as rich in calories as both pure starch and pure protein. Food, of course, is not pure fat, pure protein or pure carbohydrate, but the trend is the same. Rice and flour, for example, are about half as rich in calories as butter, and boiled potatoes are about a tenth as rich as butter. To cut down calories sensibly means eating fresh fruit and vegetables (which have as little as one-twentieth of the fat-producing effect of butter), lean meat and fish, grilled not fried, and not buttering your potatoes. Jam, chocolate, sweets are all extremely high in energy and easy to eat in large quantities, but fruit and vegetables, which are happily low in energy, give a feeling of being satisfactorily full.

Every day you should eat

- ☐ dairy produce (cheese, eggs, milk)
- ☐ meat and fish
- ☐ fruit
- ☐ vegetables
- ☐ fresh nuts
- ☐ cereals
- ☐ pulses

This will mean that you get all the vitamins, minerals, proteins, fats, and sugars as you need them, in the right sort of proportion. If you do this you will find your weight soon stabilises. Indeed, just by cutting out stodge and sugar or sweets, and reducing (not omitting) fats, you obtain a much more balanced diet, lower in calories and much healthier, too.

Another useful hint is to eat four meals a day — yes, *four*. Many fat people miss breakfast, nibble at lunch and gorge at suppertime. It is better to eat four well-balanced meals, with no temptations to nibble in between.

A good breakfast:
Cereal (vary from day to day)
Fruit (vary from day to day)
Egg or bacon or fish
Coffee/tea/fruit juice.

A good lunch:
Vegetable soup or fruit or vegetable starter
Meat or fish with unbuttered vegetables
Fruit or cheese
Dry wine
You can vary this widely.

A good tea
Fruit or wholemeal bread or vegetables.

Dinner
As for lunch, but vary such dishes as grills and boiled fish; or you can introduce nuts.

Salads of fresh vegetables with wholemeal bread make good snacks, as does fruit. Vary rice with potatoes. Try to cut out sugar altogether. Use honey if you must (honey is difficult to eat in huge quantities — it fills you up easily, unlike sugar). Avoid too much vegetable margarine, as the effect is very similar to eating too much butter.

Also, add wheatgerm to cereals (fresh not toasted), and brewers' yeast to soups, gravies and stocks. And don't forget your 4 to 7 eggs a week — they contain so many nutrients for your skin.

When drinking, remember that spirits are very rich in calories, but nothing else. Beers and stouts are rich too, but they contain some minerals. The best drink is a dry white or red wine.

THE GOOD BASKET GUIDE TO HEALTHY EATING

To help you put these ideas about food into practice, here is a guide to shopping, with further details and emphasis on important nutrients.

There are some foods which provide an energy/nutrient mix so well adapted to our needs that we should always have them. Others are so badly designed for us that we should keep away from them.

When you buy food, you are really buying carbohydrates, proteins, fats, minerals and vitamins. Briefly speaking, you use carbohydrates for energy, so that you can work; fats and proteins for repair; minerals to help your machinery keep ticking over, and vitamins to make sure it ticks over at the right speed.

The good news is that this complex list which comprises over forty different things comes already made up in very convenient packets in natural food. Otherwise, you would have to buy over forty different items.

The bad news is that many processed foods contain very few essential nutritional items.

This means that if you don't buy wisely, you will not eat properly, and although you probably won't become seriously ill, your energy and your health will suffer. In the same way, children will certainly be deprived at times, and their health will not be as good as it should be, because they are growing — in other words, building up their personal stocks of sugars, proteins, fats, minerals, and vitamins that they need for life.

Let us look at the functions of nutritional materials in a little more detail.

MINERALS

There are very many essential minerals. If you do not get them, you die. If you do not get them in the right balance, your body does not work so efficiently.

Here are just a few of the many minerals:

Mineral	Function
Magnesium	Helps the body to make its changes, especially in making energy.
Iron	Essential for making blood cells and for producing energy.
Zinc	Keeps the blood at the right degree of acidity.

Minerals are found in plentiful supply in meat, fish and dairy produce. Fresh fruit and vegetables, provided they haven't been over-processed, contain small amounts (especially of the trace elements). Wholewheat bread and whole-grain cereals are good sources too.

VITAMINS

Vitamins, like minerals, need to be eaten in the right amounts each day because we lose them through our urine. Vitamins are like jewel points in a watch, but every day we lose a jewel point, and it has to be replaced. Replacement comes from the identical vitamins that we find in our food.

Vitamin	Good source
A	Many vegetables, like carrots and tomatoes. *Comment: Important for healthy eyes and vision.*
B	Liver, seeds, grains, brown rice *Comment: There are about a dozen B vitamins; luckily they are usually found together. They are essential for the nerves, healthy skin and vitality.*
Niacin	Wheat bran, yeast *Comment: Some people appear to need greater amounts to maintain mental health.*
Riboflavin B_2	Eggs, milk *Comment: Absolutely essential for production of energy*
Folic Acid	Liver, greens *Comment: Often deficient in women*
Thiamine B_1	Yeast, whole grains *Comment: Essential for high level of energy.*
C	Fresh fruit, green vegetables and leaves. *Comment: Essential for keeping cells healthy; good for bones, ligaments and tendons. Aids resistance to infections. Smoking, oral contraceptives and stress boost the need for this vitamin.*
D	Fish, dairy produce and liver. *Comment: Necessary for growing bones and keeping bones healthy in older people.*
E	Wheat grains and plant oils. *Comment: Ensures healthy sexual development and important for healthy tissues and general fertility.*

There has recently been much talk about Pangamic acid and Vitamin C, so they deserve special assessment. Pangamic acid, B15, appears to be found wherever other vitamins of the B group are concentrated, such as seeds and especially the germ of wheat and corn. It is also found in brewers' yeast, blood and liver. Chemically it is gluconic acid, the common protein component glycine, and the very active di-isopropylamine dichloroacetate, which is known to dilate blood vessels and is therefore used in the treatment of high blood pressure.

Pangamic acid is curious because it contains chlorine atoms, unusual in vitamins, while chlorine itself, although a widely distributed and important non-metallic mineral, is with very few exceptions found in our tissues as a free charged particle, when it balances sodium particles electronically. The claims that Pangamic acid increases oxygen supply to tissues may merely be due to its increasing the size of the blood vessels.

The importance of Vitamin C is undisputed. The weight of evidence is that we should eat, not just to escape scurvy but for perfect natural functioning, at least 250 milligrams a day, which are easily obtained in oranges, fruits, greens and salads, like this:

2 oranges	60 mg
1 lb fresh potatoes	50 mg
3-4 medium tomatoes	100 mg

The balance can be made up from greens, fruits, vegetables, berries, melons, pineapples, tomatoes.

In winter, a 100 mg per day supplement of Vitamin C is a good idea.

These are just a few of the undisputed vitamins. All of them are deficient in over-refined, over-cooked and underbalanced diets.

If, on checking the way you eat, the above foods do not figure every day in your diet, you need to improve your regime. But you should never try to make up your vitamin deficiencies in your diet by eating pills because: the mix and balance of B vitamins is not understood; the balance in natural foods is probably nearer the mix we require than any other formulation; we cannot be sure that pills of 100, or even 10,000, times the potency of natural mixes have no serious effects over a long period.

It follows then, that there are no wonder vitamins or nutrients to keep you in perfect health. Your diet is the foundation of your health.

If you are overweight, smoke heavily, take no exercise, drink in excess and worry, you are deluding yourself if you think popping any pill, whether drug or vitamin, will do much to put right these ravages.

PROTEINS

The proteins we eat are made up of about twenty different units: the amino acids. Some proteins contain all the amino acids in a good mixture, but synthetic proteins are often low on some acids, and so cannot entirely substitute for meat. Cereals, when mixed, give a good balance too, but taken singly often have one, or even two essential acids in too low a supply. First-class proteins are cheese, fish, eggs, meat.

FATS

Apart from the figure-forming function of

fat in the skin, fat also surrounds the nerves and is essential to their healthy functioning. A balanced mixture of fats, such as those found in meat and butter, and lipids, the high-quality mixed fats, to be found in egg yolk, liver, nuts and plant oils, is essential.

Generally, you can stay healthy and go a long way towards escaping illness by avoiding food that contains additives or synthetic vitamins, and by eating a sound diet.

This takes a great deal of time. It means shopping with care, and eschewing all junk foods. The general rule is: eat fresh, eat varied, eat small, and eat often.

Why is our diet today so bad and so destructive? The answer is extraordinarily simple: we have been over-successful in food production in the West, and now we are processing it. We evolved—that is to say, were designed—by eating a wide mix of fresh food. We used to spend most of our time finding food, and eating it. At first, although even then recognisably men and women, we obtained most of our energy from plant foods, of which we had to eat huge amounts to get sufficient energy to survive, but in so doing we also took in large amounts of minerals and vitamins, in a wide variety. When we became more successful in hunting, calories came increasingly from meat—fresh meat. Calculations show, without much room for doubt, that all the vitamins in such a diet, at its best, were several times higher than we get today and, in the case of vitamin C, the factor is nearer a hundred times higher.

What, then, are the good foods, and what are the bad?

The basic list is: dairy produce, meats and fish, cereals, fruits, vegetables. Something of each of these should figure every day in your diet.

BUT:

always choose traditional cheese rather than processed

never buy boiled milk

buy meat from a butcher, not in cans (corned beef for instance, is often saturated with sugar)

buy fresh fruit and vegetables.

Particularly good common foods are: the potato—an excellent mix of the nutrients, and it is not energy-saturated unless dripping in frying fat; milk; eggs; liver; nuts (fresh, not roasted and salted).

A good shopping basket (add up all the shopping baskets for the separate days of the week) and a bad basket to be avoided would be:

GOOD BASKET

Wholewheat breads and buns, fresh eggs, milk, cheese, lean butchers' meat, liver, fresh (or good frozen) fish, tinned pilchards, sardines, fresh peas, beans; fresh greens, salads, fresh potatoes, apples, oranges, bananas, some butter, plant oils for frying, honey for concentrated energy, good quality jams, dried fruits for minerals and energy, wholegrain cereals.

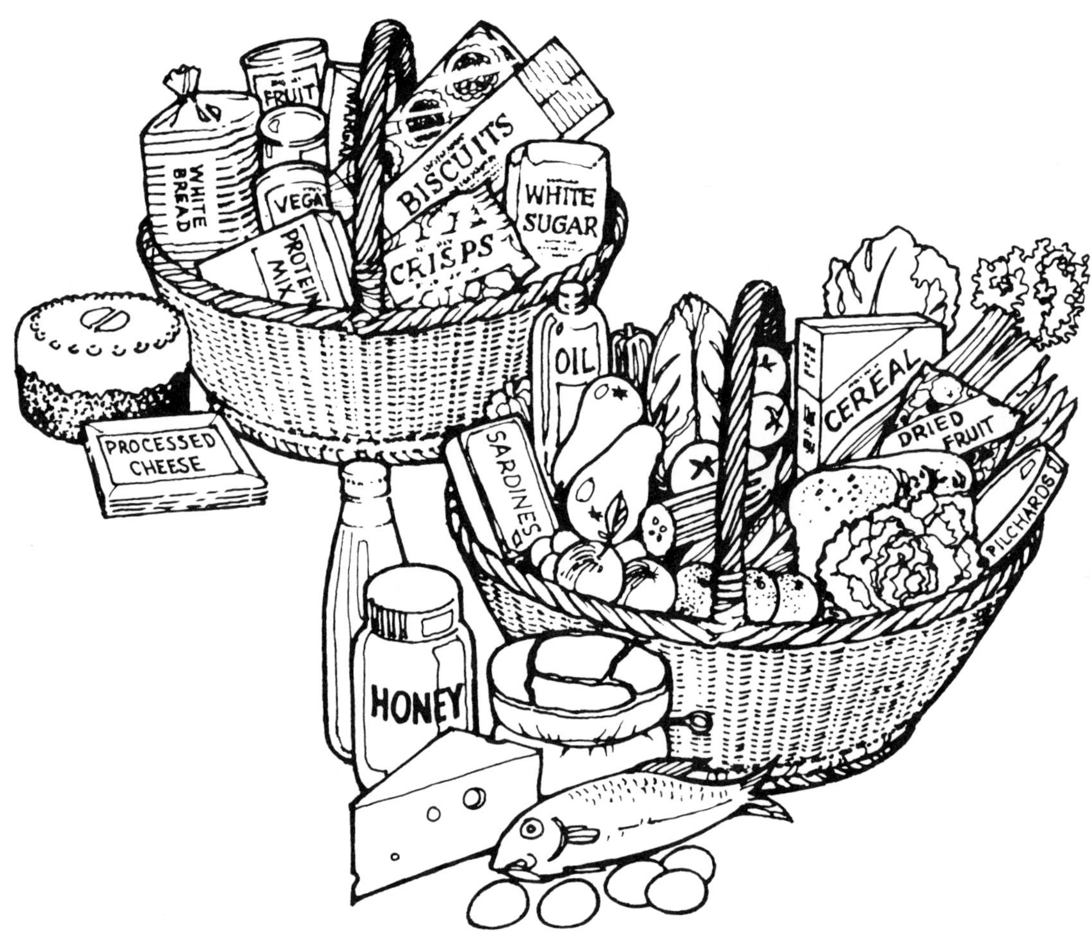

BAD BASKET

White bread, tinned vegetables, tinned fruits, synthetic protein mixes, crisps, biscuits, cakes, excessive amounts of vegetable oils and margarines, white rice, white flour, processed cheeses, white sugar (brown is just as bad).

What about the cost? Even today you can buy fresh fruit and vegetables more cheaply than their processed equivalents, but you need to spend time on their preparation. Meat is not excessively expensive if you avoid buying prime steak; and the cheaper, coarser cuts make excellent stews for the winter, and fill up any voracious child or man properly. Cheese, which remains a first-class investment for your basket, is a good energy food and nutritionally rich. Milk, too, is cheap for the food value it contains; while the foods in the bad basket may fill a mouth, may fill a tummy, but they won't fill the bones, brain or blood with proper nutrients.

If you are not convinced, the next time you are in the supermarket look at overweight people and see what they are buying, or pick out someone who looks really trim and healthy, and have a look at his or her basket. It won't work every time, of course, because age and other factors operate, but in general you'll see the good signs go with a good basket, and the bad with the bad basket.

Chapter Three

SWIMMING

SWIMMING

Swimming is a wonderful way of exercising your body. The basic swimming strokes utilise a great many muscles which are often neglected by other sports and exercise routines. In this chapter you will find the four basic strokes and their variations. It is important to learn these as they form the basis for the special water exercises that follow and will give you confidence in the water.

When your body is immersed in water it is supported and becomes virtually weightless: consequently it is possible to do exercise of a very moderate kind. Also, by using the fact that the water resistance increases rapidly the harder you push against it, you can do extremely high rates of exercise. This makes swimming and work in the water much more suitable for people who haven't been exercising well than, for example, taking up jogging.

For the very fit person, water resistance—pushing against the water with your limbs and body—increases as the effort increases, and consequently you can never really exhaust the possibilities. If you are overweight and unfit you can begin the exercises in this book in a very gentle manner and therefore avoid putting a huge strain on the heart, which in so many cases proves fatal.

On the other hand, because the water supports you, you can identify the particular muscles you want to exercise. Also, by working in water and using the exercises in this book gently, you can gradually increase the strength of your muscles, and as they become stronger they will be able to do more work, and the heart can follow.

Jogging is extremely bad for any figure-conscious woman. The pounding of feet on hard, city streets is not good for the ankles, not good for the knees and not good for the hips. It imposes unnecessary strain upon muscles and ligaments, stretching them, pulling them and, in some cases, even breaking small bones, while the poor heart is suddenly called upon to do five or six times its normal amount of work. This is a recipe for discomfort at least and, as any doctor will tell you, often a recipe leading to far more serious results.

It is true that with exercise the body becomes stronger and the heart will also become stronger. But it is best to take the exercise gently over a longish period of time: quite frankly, I do not believe in programmes of the kind that are in vogue now. You should ask yourself whether or not what you are doing feels bad. If it feels bad and you have to make a huge effort, it is not doing you good at all. It is doing you harm. You should have no sensation of distress, no sensation of pain. My exercises, the ones on land and also on water, as described here, give pleasure and they are so developed and so graded that you can gradually work your way up at your own pace, becoming better and better and stronger and stronger.

Swimming is quite natural to us. It is only fear imbued in childhood that stops most people learning very quickly. People tell children, quite rightly, that they mustn't go near water, and they don't, so they become frightened of it. The right part of this is the warning of the possible danger of water. The wrong part is that nothing has been done to allay the fear. One should treat water with respect. If you haven't been able to learn to swim, the best thing is to go to a swimming-bath and, at the shallow end, see if you can float. All you have to do is push your chest out by breathing deeply and you will find you can float quite well. Relax: stop being tense and your body will become supple.

If you can't swim, it's as well to find someone who can show you. Although it is not essential (many of the routines require only a shallow depth of water) a knowledge of basic swimming strokes will help you considerably, and aid your confidence and expertise in the water.

If you can swim, now follows an analysis of the figure-forming and exercise benefits of certain strokes. In **1** and **2** you see the basic over-arm and splashing of the legs of a very heavy crawl. When you bend the legs up as shown, you exercise the outer thigh and the front of the thigh. This kind of motion is excellent for the legs, the back and the arms. Notice how the breathing is shown in **2**, where by the forward push through the water there is usually a wave underneath the cheek that enables you to breathe well. However, it is possible to do the crawl in a more leisurely way where you never kick up so

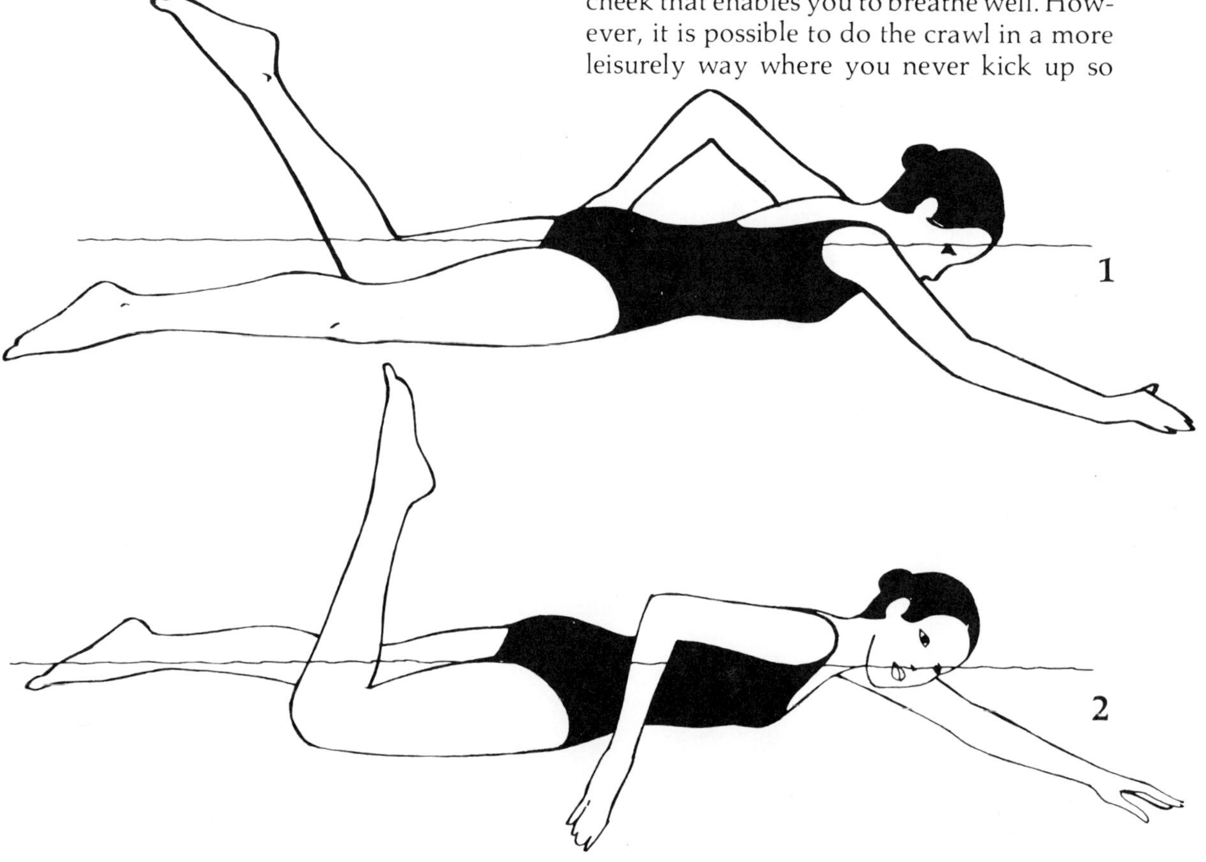

high but keep the legs more or less straight and move them at the hips. This movement is good for the hips and gives lean shapely legs. The kicking technique often produces a very fast type of swim but it will shorten the muscles rather than lengthen them. Also, when doing the crawl you must reach out with the arms in order to get a good line in the back. This is particularly beneficial for the muscles underneath the breasts and gives a good line. However, beware of doing too much crawling because it does emphasise the front of the thighs and the chest muscles. If this is your only style you will develop huge chest muscles, though it is marvellous if you want to increase your bust size.

In **3** and **4** you see the basic shape for the breast-stroke, and here you are using different sets of muscles. You are working on the inside of the thighs rather than the outside, and the outside of the chest rather than the front of the chest. This is a good exercise if you do it very easily and gracefully, kicking with your legs and sweeping your arms round in an arc through the water in time, as shown in sequence **3** and **4.** The curious thing about the breast-stroke is that no matter how slowly you do it you will stay afloat and breathe quite easily and nicely, whereas with the crawl there is a certain minimum speed below which you begin to lose control and get the idea you are sinking. Therefore, for long-distance swimming, people often use the breast-stroke. When done very energetically, it has the good effect of stretching the back of the arms and the inside of the thighs with a slimming result in these areas, but, of course, if you do it very hard you will build more muscle.

With the backstroke shown in the sequence

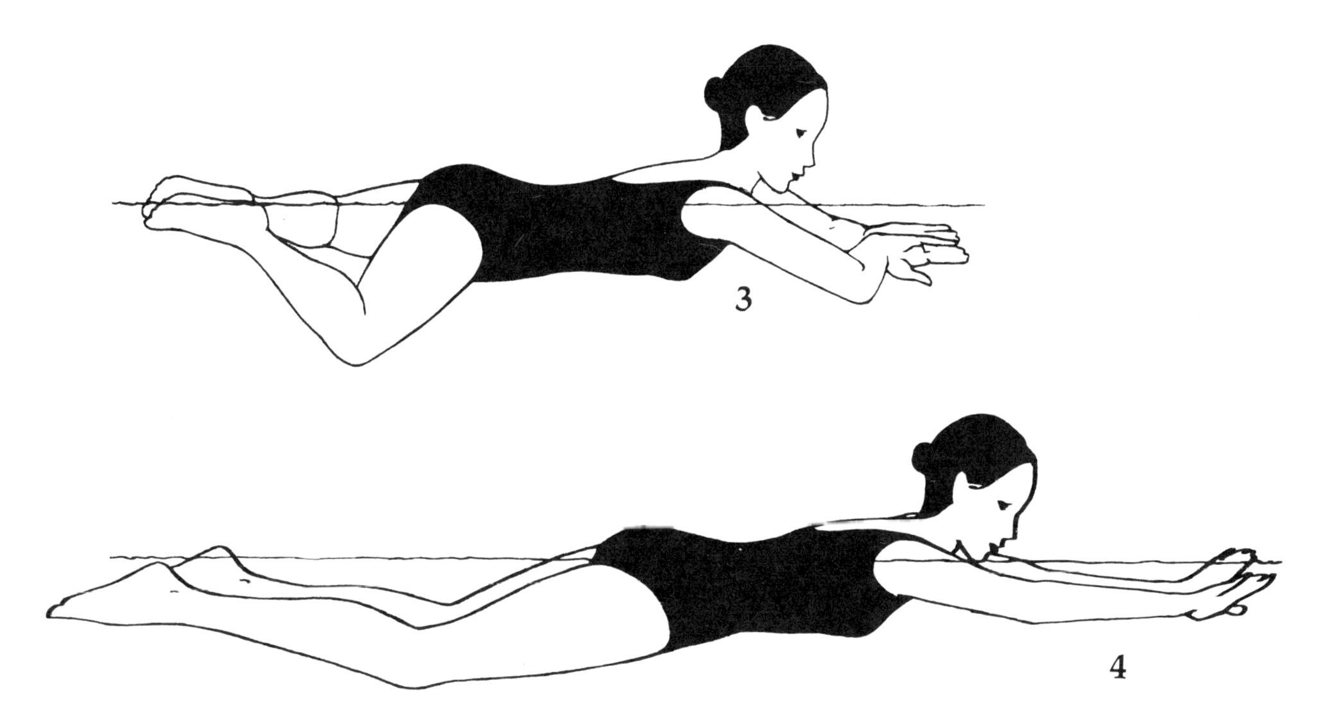

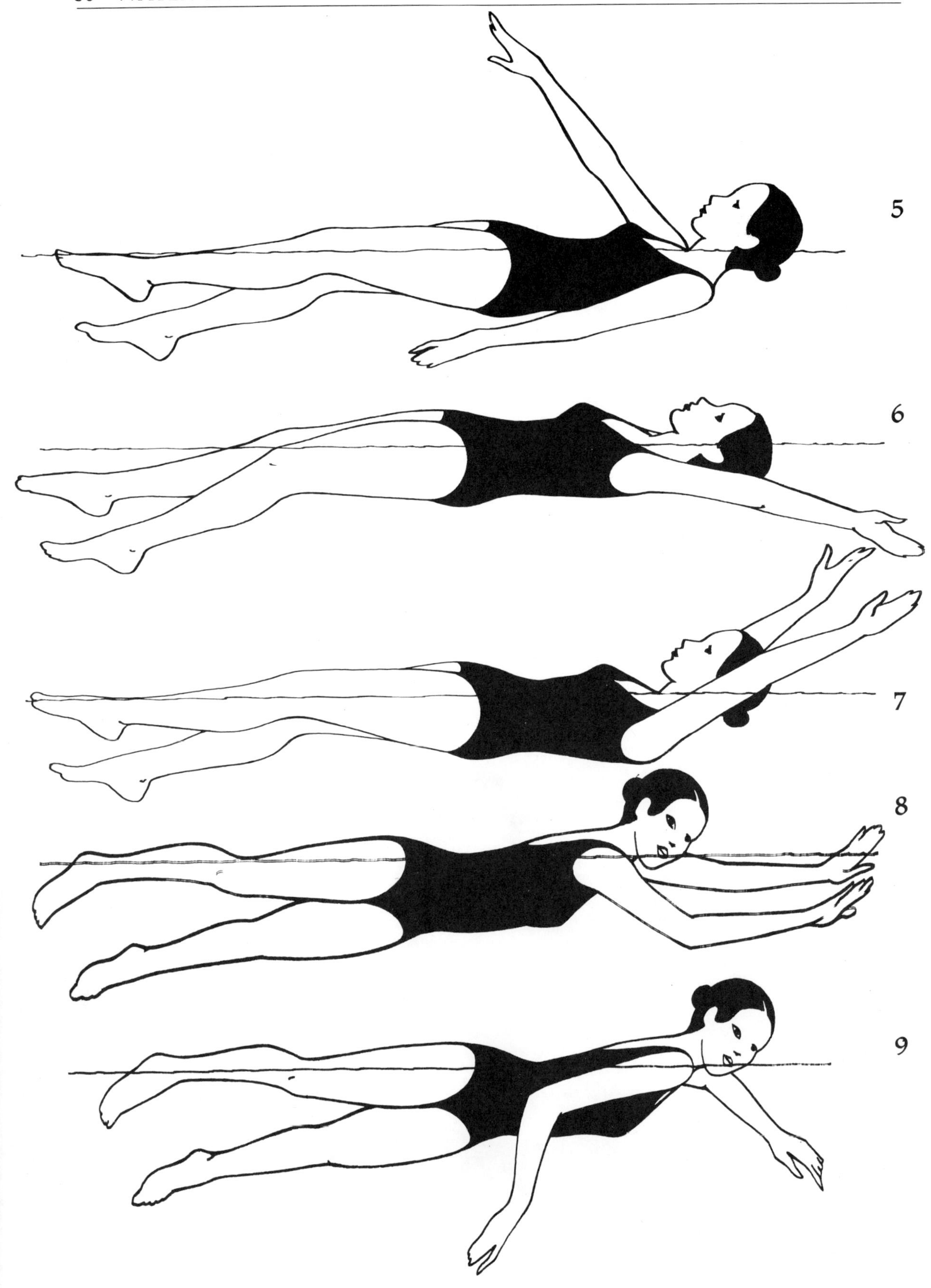
5
6
7
8
9

5 and **6** there is alternate raising and lowering. This is excellent for a good line in the waist and also nice long muscles in the legs. It is a marvellous figure-former, and the relaxing movements are good for the head muscles, the shoulder muscles and the neck. You can vary it a little by using both arms as shown in **7**. It is much more energetic but has basically the same effect as **5** and **6**.

A beautiful stroke is the side-stroke, a variation of which is shown in **8** and **9**. The great thing about this is the exercise of one side of the body at a time.

If you are really interested in building up a beautifully balanced figure then you should do each of the strokes very relaxedly for about 50 yards: that is 50 yards of crawl, 50 yards of breast-stroke, 50 yards of backstroke and 50 yards of side-stroke. Do one after the other, taking it very easily; then have a rest. This will help towards an over-all development of the body which, in conjunction with the specialist work later on in the book, will help you build up a superb figure.

Keep on looking in the mirror as the days go by, seeing which parts of your body are improving and which parts are improving rather less, then pick out the right exercise in the book for your specific needs and concentrate on that.

I am very much in favour of children learning to do all four strokes because they form a very good over-all exercise. Children should never be given stereotyped exercise, such as doing only the breast-stroke or only the crawl. This leads to distortion of the figure—as anyone can see from those unfortunate girls from East Germany who have been turned into robots by doing one particular kind of swimming. I think if you observe their figures that my points about the bad effects of unvaried kinds of swimming are borne out. A gold medal is never going to compensate for distorted muscles or rib-cages caused by performing the wrong kind of exercise for too long a time. Children, then, should be encouraged to do all of the strokes. When your bones stop growing—in girls this is about 16-17 years of age, in boys 18-19—then you can start working on specific parts of the body to obtain the right kind of shape for your particular figure type.

PERFORMANCE GRADINGS FOR SWIMMERS

	100 metres free style Optimum (seconds)	Fit	Medium
Up to 35			
Men	53	80	100
Women	60	90	120
35-55			
Men	58	95	120
Women	66	110	130
55+			
Men	64	110	130
Women	73	125	140

The Optimum performances are beyond most people, while the Fit may be reasonably aimed at, over a period of time. The Medium performances are very good for older people, but for younger groups, remember that to get in the water and swim 100 metres, even in 150 seconds, is infinitely better than not doing it at all. In swimming, technique is very important. The aim here is to get you thinking about what you can do.

PERFORMANCE SCHEDULES FOR LONGER DISTANCES

	Up to 35		35+	
	Men	Women	Men	Women
1500 metres free-style Optimum (minutes)	16	17	18	19

The Optimum performances are beyond most people. Try adding five, even fifteen, minutes to the above times, and see how you can work down during the year.

SAFETY IN THE WATER

Many people get cramp, often because they go into water that is too deep or too cold. For instance, at 4°C (39°F) even a strong, experienced swimmer cannot expect to stand the stress for more than about ten minutes. The ability to withstand coldness without special training goes down to about three or four minutes at 0°C (32°F). So, always try to swim in warm water. There is nothing clever about breaking ice and jumping into icy water.

Always avoid letting children go swimming by themselves. There are far too many lives lost in inland waterways. Many teenagers and adults in their twenties die by drowning in the sea, often through being foolhardy, forgetting how strong the sea is and going out of their depth. Curiously, more men drown than women. This may have something to do with their desire to show off, or it may be due to the fact that women have more natural fat in their bodies and so can withstand the cold better. Do not think that you can drink alcohol and safely go into the sea or swimming-pool. In Australia, one person in five who has been drowned has a high level of alcohol in his blood. In Scotland, it is almost one person in three. The reason, apparently, is not merely befuddlement of the senses but a biochemical fact that muscular exercise, after an excessive intake of alcohol, reduces the amount of sugar in the blood and often leads to a coma.

There is some mystery about the fact that people can appear to have been drowned, immersed in water, for up to ten minutes yet have survived. Usually, when a person lacks oxygen, the brain expires after about three minutes. When a person is drowning there is some mechanism in the body, often called the diving reflex which enables the brain to keep functioning, but the details are obscure. The practical effect of this means that if you are ever in this situation, you should never give up early in trying to resuscitate somebody. The drowned person may appear dead, but with skilful life-saving techniques and mouth-to-mouth resuscitation, they can still be brought round even though they may have been unconscious for many minutes.

Finally, there are some points regarding safety that should never be forgotten. When you are swimming in unknown water, always ask local people about it. Always find out about currents, tide and temperature. Ask about special features—whether there are poisonous fish or plants there. Always proceed with some caution, don't just dive in. You do not know what is underneath the surface. Can you see the bottom? What about rocks, and so forth? Never swim long distances in totally unknown water. The strongest swimmer can be exhausted by currents. Get to know the area. Remember that objects that look close over water are often very much further away, so make sure. Ask yourself, can you be certain to make that dinghy, that shore, that rock, that boat? They're often not as near as you think. If you haven't swum in the sea very much, and I mean not a mere 200 yards out from the shore but several miles be warned. The first time you ever try it, the sudden realisation that you are miles away from land, that there are probably several hundred feet of water underneath you, and that even a slight breeze can produce waves that tower fifteen to twenty feet above you, making you feel terribly small, can have a greatly panicking effect, even on the stoutest heart.

Do be careful about boats. People in boats often zoom about at great speeds and they do not see you until after they've hit you! Every beach has a horror story of someone being chopped up alive.

Chapter Four

SPECIFIC FIGURE PLANS

SPECIFIC FIGURE PLANS

To get the best out of your exercises you need to know your physique type. There are four main types of bodies for women and four for men, and each type has special strengths and special weaknesses, which if known to you early enough can save you a lot of time and money. Time: because you know what you can aim for—realistically. Money: because you can cut down your medical and clothes bills by staying healthy and slim.

Our bodies are made of bone, muscles, fat and skin, with soft tissues like the liver and fluids like blood. The thinnest kind of skeleton, with very thin muscles and thin skin, is one kind of extreme physique. Another kind is when the bones are large, the muscles large, the fat little. Another is large bones, smallish muscles, lots of fat, all in perfect proportion as in a Greek god or goddess; then there is the fourth kind of extreme: a perfectly balanced physique.

Below are check lists of the main types of physique, the slim, muscular and rounded builds. You can assess to a fair degree of accuracy what type you are from these trait lists.

THE SLIM BUILD

- thin bones
- stringy muscles
- very thin on side view
- long limbs in comparison to length of trunk
- prominent but thin ribs
- narrow shoulders
- little muscle on body
- marked hollow behind collar-bone
- long forearms and shins in comparison to upper part of limbs
- fragile fingers and toes, thin joints, not prominent but little and pointed
- long neck
- fragile-looking skull, not rounded
- thin skin
- skin does not tan easily
- little elasticity in skin (a pinch takes time to return to original position)

THE NATURALLY MUSCULAR BUILD

- strong square body
- clearly defined muscles
- very strongly made wrists and ankles
- strongly made and strongly jointed feet and fingers

strong and large joints
prominent muscular buttocks
clear and rippling tummy muscles
thick and strongly made ribs
low waist
conspicuous pores
thick and strong tendons

THE LARGE ROUNDED BUILD

round soft body
width and depth in limbs tend to be the same (round thighs, round ankle and wrist, round calf)
the upper parts of the limbs very much bigger than the extremities
short neck
very smooth body contours
abdominal muscles not clearly defined
the bones of wrist and ankle, knee and elbow do not project
on feeling, smooth, round bones, especially joints; collar bone not clearly seen
smooth rib-cage
soft, smooth, velvety skin

The perfectly balanced physique has strong but not rugged joints; muscles that are smooth and not over-conspicuous; fat under the skin no thicker than half an inch in women, and about three-eighths of an inch in men. Very few people are exactly like this, but a slight majority of people have more nearly a balanced mixture of thin—plus rounded—plus muscular build than any other combination. We call this the average physique because it is so general.

Put in perspective, we see that women of the muscular type are much more rounded than men of this type, while slim women are often smooth and soft in comparison to their male counterparts. Rounded women are, of course, much more usual than rounded men. Women of all four types have larger hips than chests and much less muscle, weight for weight, than similar males. The following table showing representative values for bodily measurements at 5 feet 6 inches for women and 5 feet 9 inches for men will help to focus these types.

BUILD IN INCHES

	Slim		Balanced		Muscular		Rounded	
	Men	Women	Men	Women	Men	Women	Men	Women
Chest (bust for women)	34	34	38	35½	41	37	41	39
Waist	27	26	29	27	30	29	35	32
Hips	34	36	36	38	39	39½	41	42

These values go up in direct proportion for taller heights, down for shorter. You can see how much smaller the chests of women are, because the bust measurement includes the breasts. The waists are measured with tummy let out *not* pulled in.

The values are of men and women who are not overweight, but who are not developed as well as they could be by exercise.

Now that you have a good idea of your body type, you can use the knowledge best by checking off your needs in the schedules below.

COMMON FIGURE AND HEALTH PROBLEMS

Slim build: there is a tendency to stoop because the muscles are not strong. Women lose curves because the skin gets too thin. Overweight is never a problem with this build, but the waist can sag through neglect.
Balanced build: overweight is often to be found: two or three inches on the waist, three to four on the hips are very common conditions.
Muscular build: same as *Balanced*, but the weight increase is even bigger.
Rounded build: incredibly the 41-35-41 man easily blows up to 42-50-50, while the woman blows up from 39-32-42 to 43-50-53 in extreme cases.

THE AIMS OF THE BODY TYPES ARE:

Women

Slim type:	to produce smoother lines
Balanced:	to strengthen waist, smooth hips
Muscular:	to maintain weight and good line
Rounded:	to make muscles strong to keep shape

Men

Slim type:	to strengthen body and maintain weight
Balanced:	to strengthen abdominal muscles
Muscular:	to maintain weight and muscle tone
Rounded:	to develop muscles, reduce excess fat

Pregnancy

Ideally, water exercises make you very strong and fit, so that when you become pregnant you will not have the same troubles as women who are not fit. This is chiefly because you will have improved your diet, and because your muscles are so much stronger and well exercised that they will more easily adapt to your changing shape.

In pregnancy, as at any other time of life when starting exercises after a period of neglect, do not begin with too much vigour. If you have already been doing water exercises it is beneficial to continue them during pregnancy, bearing the following points in mind:

You should do all the exercises you like, but cut down the intensity and effort; always do them very gently. As your pregnancy advances, you should do them even more slowly and carefully. You should, of course, avoid diving and jumping from the very onset. Gentle movements, flowing and graceful, will do you and your growing baby a lot of good.

As you become heavier, you will find that the buoyancy of the water supports you and helps you to feel lighter so that you can concentrate on your movements.

Water exercises will also improve your breathing and the supply of oxygen in your blood which is essential for the developing baby.

Very slim women tend to get tired easily during pregnancy, so the relaxing effect of lying in water is particularly beneficial. Athletic and curvaceous women tend to put on far too much weight during pregnancy. Gentle swimming will help to restore the balance. Women of average build usually experience less extreme reactions, but they often become overtired and overweight, so a gentle exercise routine is beneficial.

After the baby is born you will need to take medical advice for your personal needs. Provided you consult your doctor or clinic about what you intend to do, there is every reason why you should continue exercising.

You must never try violent exercise, jogging or rough sports. Exercise is to strengthen and shape you.

There are areas you need to work on. Remember, gently does it; patiently, regularly and intelligently. The waist, tummy and hips need gently persuasive care. Study the sequences under these headings and pick out by experiment the ones you like. You will need to work on your legs, too.

The gentle stroking massage methods are useful during pregnancy, but do not exert too much pressure. After the birth you can use massage techniques with progressive intensity so that you are back to normal exercise routines in six months.

Four Basic Shaping Exercises

Whatever your build, whether you are male or female, fit or fat, these four basic exercises form an excellent warming-up routine and introduction to the specific figure plans.

Start gently and work up to a longer period of time. Check your pulse rates and see how they go up and how quickly they recover. Don't overdo it; a sense of strain is not what one wants, but the good feeling the work-out gives you, and the confidence you get as you feel your heart rates gradually settle at a lower level for the same performance, and recover more and more quickly.

THE WATER ENGINE

Stand upright in water up to your waist with the feet wide apart. **1:** put your hands, palms forward, behind the back of your neck. Now squat right down, keeping your back entirely straight. Press hard with the palms of your hands, with your fingers interlocked. **2:** propel yourself rapidly out of the water as high as you can, **3.**

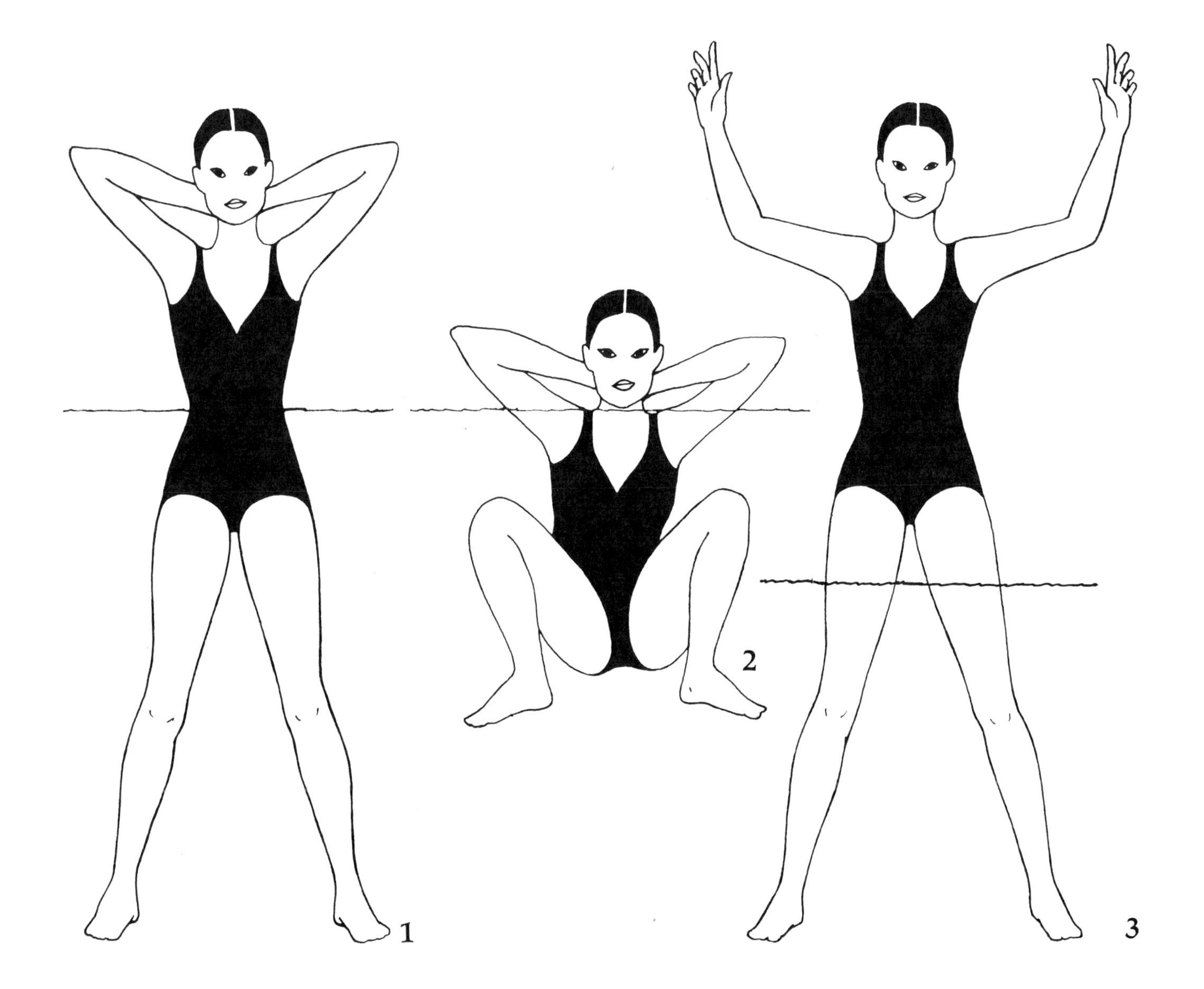

THE TWISTER

Stand erect with your legs about 18 inches apart in water halfway between crotch and navel. **4:** keeping your feet still, and without moving your shoulders, rotate your pelvis first to the right and then to the left, as far as you can. **5:** the aim here is to make your hips work against the water like a paddle, back and forth.

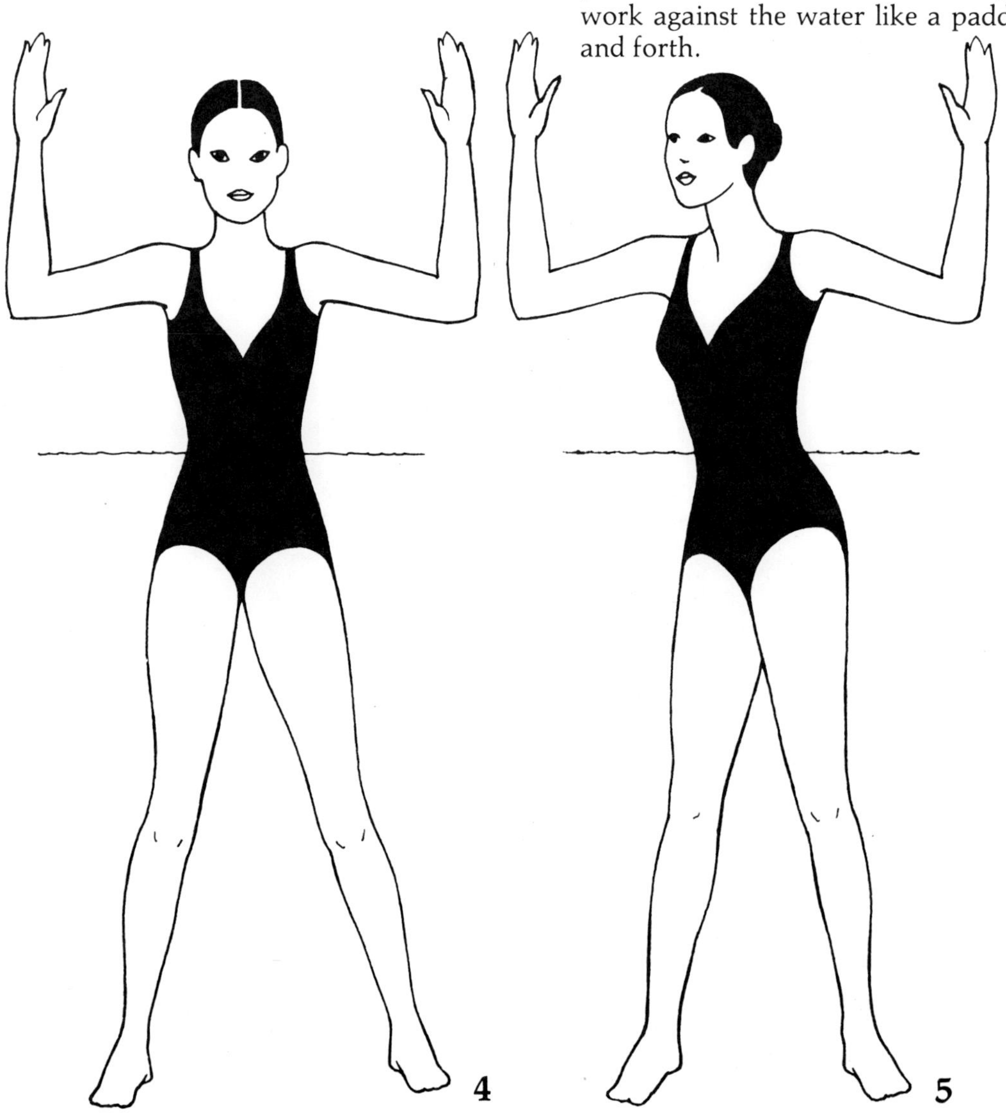

THE PADDLE

Start as with 'the twister' but, this time, push your pelvis forward and then back. The aim is to push against the water and then retreat into it, **6.**

THE TURBINE

Take up 'the twister' position. Bend forward, arms out, knees bent, and sway your hips around to the left as far as you can, and then to the right, **7.**

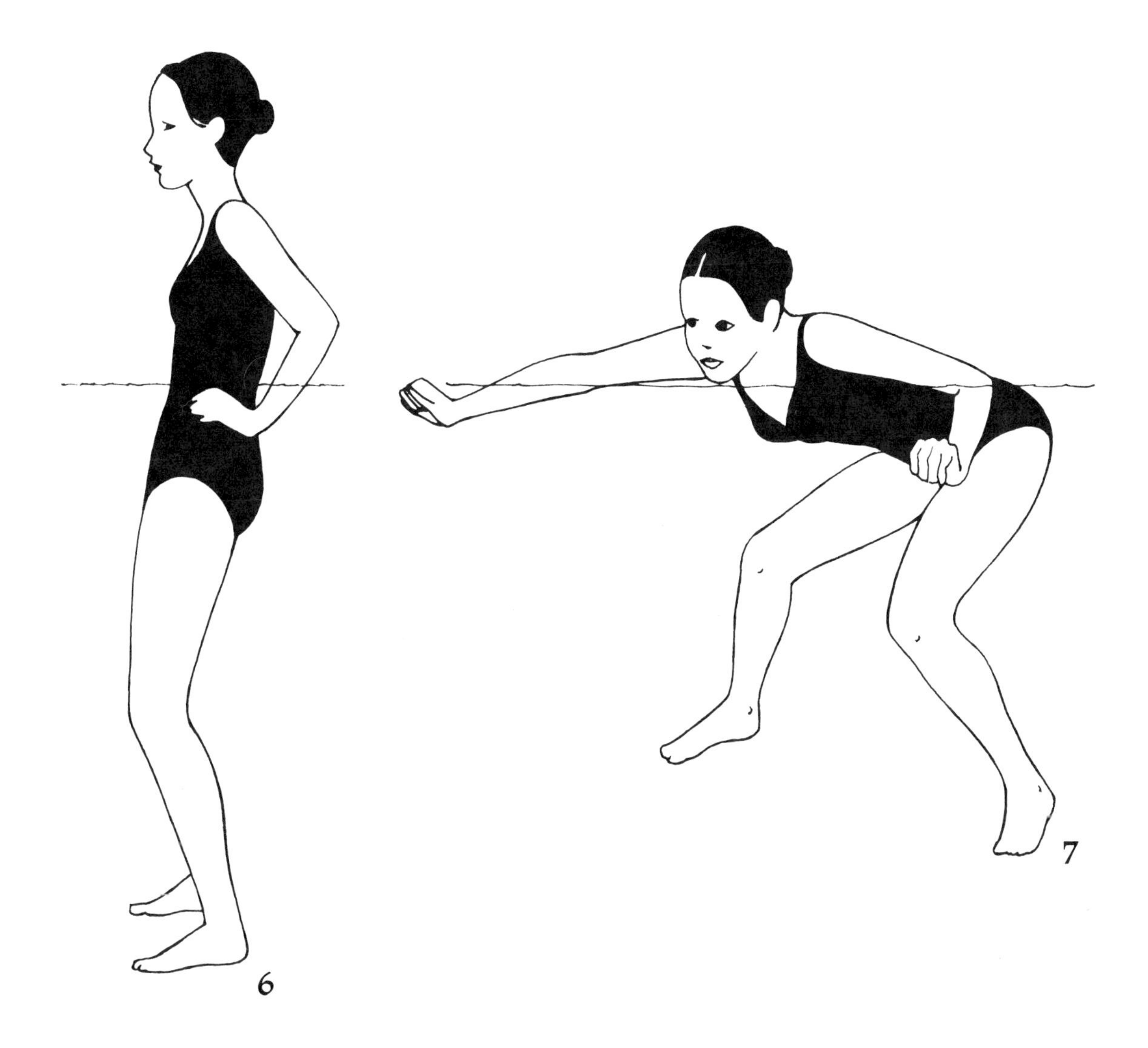

THE FOUR BASIC SHAPING EXERCISES

		Schedules (No. of times to be performed)	
Movement	**Shapes**	**Beginners**	**Advanced**
The water engine	Back, legs	3	10
The twister	Waist, hips	10	20
The paddle	Waist, small of back	12	25
The turbine	Back, waist	10	30

These are a good start to shaping your body. Men who wish to build up muscle should work up to Advanced and then go on to do the whole sequence of exercises at one time, rest, and repeat. In general you should start by working over your whole body, then concentrate on the parts you want to shape and slim by working through the appropriate schedules in the book.

If you want to use the exercises to slim, perform them more quickly, but with the minimum of resistance in the water, which will mean you use a minimum depth for your body. For example, when performing the arm exercises, your arm can be only a few inches in the water, and so not meet much resistance. If, however, you want to build tissue, perhaps if you are very slim and angular, you gradually build up your weight by eating well, as I explained, and use the greatest depth of water, so that you have more water to move against, and perform the exercise as hard as you can.

The general principle is: light effort with great speed is slimming: great effort, performed as hard as possible (it will be slow because of the water resistance), will build up tissue.

Men who wish to develop a strong body can do so by following the above principles, and women will find that they can develop superbly shaped and supple bodies, without any evidence of excessive bulging muscles at all, by using the standard exercises in the depth of water described.

Chapter Five

LEGS

LEGS

Legs are pre-eminently important in a good figure and healthy body because they carry the weight and work so hard. They also complete the line of the body.

Women have naturally curving thighs that continue their line to the waist, which being much narrower than the hips gives a profoundly feminine shape. Unfortunately, this natural female shape is often spoiled by the thighs where excess weight is most easily deposited.

The shape of the leg depends on a good muscle line, and that can only be achieved and maintained by exercising all the muscles in a balanced way, particularly the long muscles on the outside, front and insides of the thighs which have to be strong.

These exercises will help to give you a firm layer on top of the muscles as well as stimulating the blood flow and regulating the natural layer of fat. They will also ensure that the ankle, the knee and the hip joints are properly exercised—so important for keeping them supple and for posture.

You cannot do much about your bone structure, but you can shape and strengthen your legs; ensure that the muscles are in good tone, and that the fat layer is adequately thick and, like the skin, smooth.

TONE

Feel your legs while sitting cross-legged without clothes on. Feel the inside of your thighs, underneath them, outside, by pinching and pressing with your fingertips. Now do the same to your calves. If you can feel hard, knotted muscles, they are in bad tone. You can help them by massage, preferably after a bath, using a moisturising cream. Follow the sequences shown in the drawings in Chapters Nine and Ten, noting the position of the hands and body. At first, you may find that some are difficult because your muscles are over-contracted. This is really hard work.

SHAPE

For building up under-developed legs, several months are necessary to give shape, and the exercises are time-consuming but they do give smoothness of contour. What is needed is a gradual stimulus to the whole leg tissue by increasing the blood flow. Do these exercises very slowly.

Study the drawings carefully, and read the instructions just as carefully. Don't rush it—in time the exercises will become second nature. The secret of success lies in the gentle increase of contraction of the muscle.

SKIN

Rub body cream or oil into your legs once a week. Do not forget your improved diet, because your nutrition may be inadequate, and only with a balanced diet can you have beauty and health.

These exercises can be done in a swimming-bath at the shallow end, with your hands on the rail behind you, or on the beach in water 1-2 feet deep.

Ankles and Knees

THE GYROSCOPE

For shaping and strengthening ankles and knees, take position **1** and gradually extend the leg to position **2** keeping the toes pointed at all times. Now bring the leg back up to position **1** again. A variation is to perform 'the gyroscope' but with the legs open, which has more effect on the upper thighs.

Calves

The calves, these days, are more or less on constant show. They are also very hard worked, bearing, as they do, most of the weight of the body. It is not surprising that they reveal very quickly whether or not they are being looked after.

Too much walking in excessively high heels shortens the calf muscles, and the sharp persistent thumping they get while absorbing the whole weight of the body in each step, in day-to-day work on hard surfaces, accentuates a bunching effect. The result is a thickening of the ankle, often due to fluid, and a loss of curvaceous line. My exercises in water elongate the muscles, making them smoother and more elastic, and put them through more of the movements they were

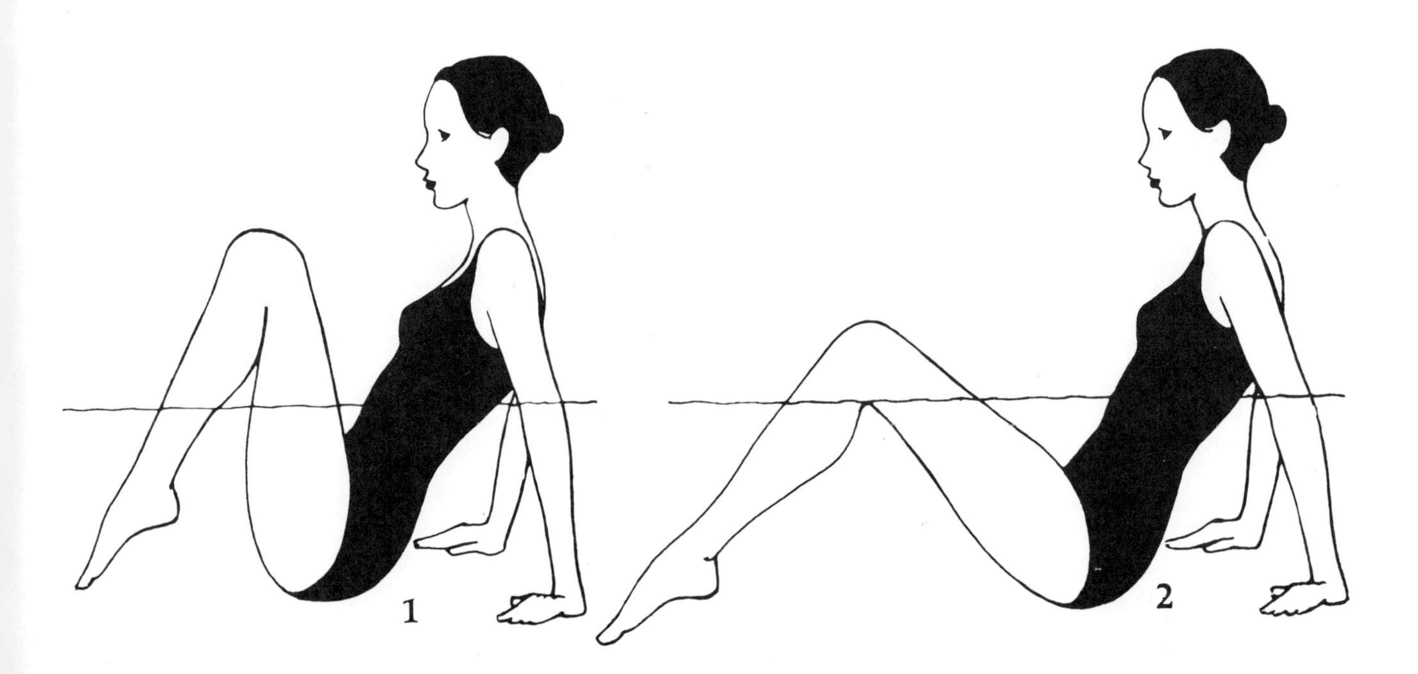

designed to perform than they get by simply walking.

Long hours of standing put pressure on the blood vessels. Blood returns upwards from the toes, up the leg, partly as the result of a pumping action by the muscles. So to guard against distention of veins leading to unsightly bulges, exercise in water, thereby freeing the muscles from weight yet actively encouraging blood flow. This helps to build up resistance to the deleterious effects I have described.

In addition to the exercises shown here, try the massage methods too, making sure you work up from the ankle towards the knee. Don't forget your shins as there are muscles there as well. You will soon discover how your muscles (hard and knotted, which no muscle should be), soon respond to the gentle persuasion of massage and exercise.

THE WAVE

The simple exercise shown in **3** involves the following movements: start as shown, toes pointed. Then force the legs down into the water until they reach the same level as the knees **4.** Now raise them rapidly to the starting position again. Repeat until you feel a very tiny ache in the calf. Then point your toes away from you, feet in the right-angled position as if you were walking on them. Curl the toes up, and repeat the movement. After a while you will be able to vary the angle of the ankle, working against the water pressure with your sole and the top surface of your feet.

A variation of this exercise is to hold on to the side of the swimming-bath, where you will get much heavier exercise of the calf muscles; or you can have someone hold your hands in the sea.

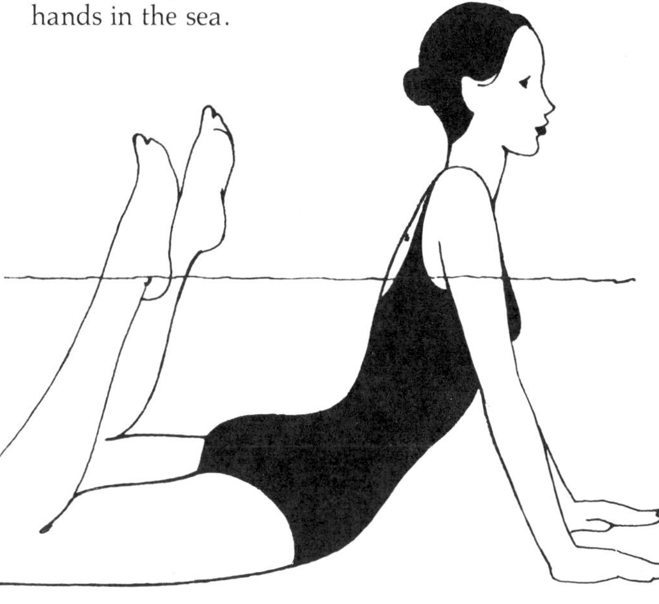

3

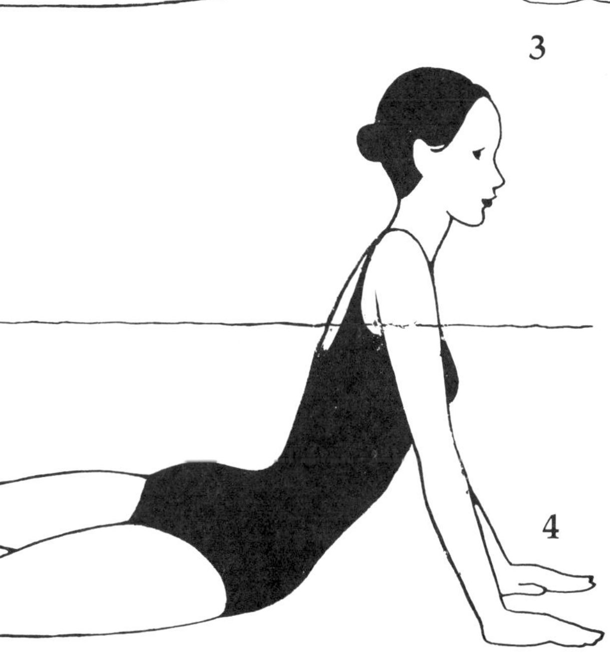

4

Thighs

THE CLAM

For the inside of the thighs put the feet together, the soles firmly pressed, as shown in position **5.** Now let the legs fall under their own weight through the water as shown in **6,** and then bring them up sharply against the water weight so that your thighs touch as shown in drawing **7.** Press them back down to position **6.** This exercises the inside and outside of the thighs; areas which often get deposits of fat.

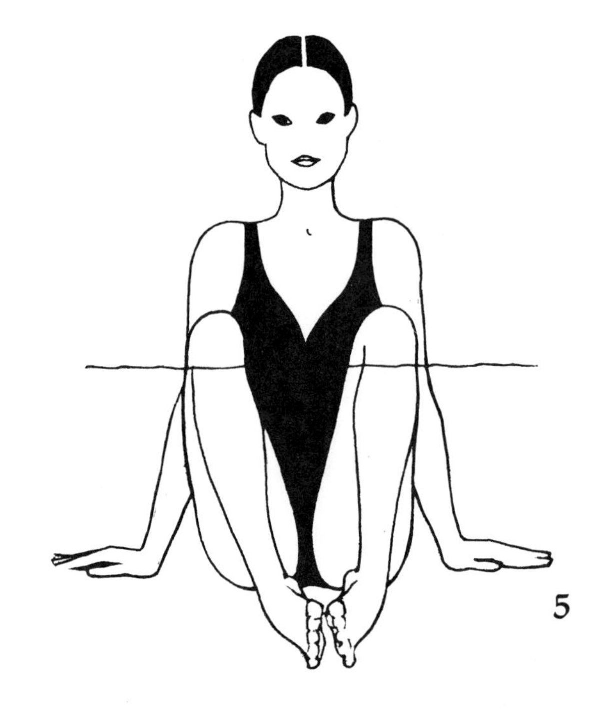

5

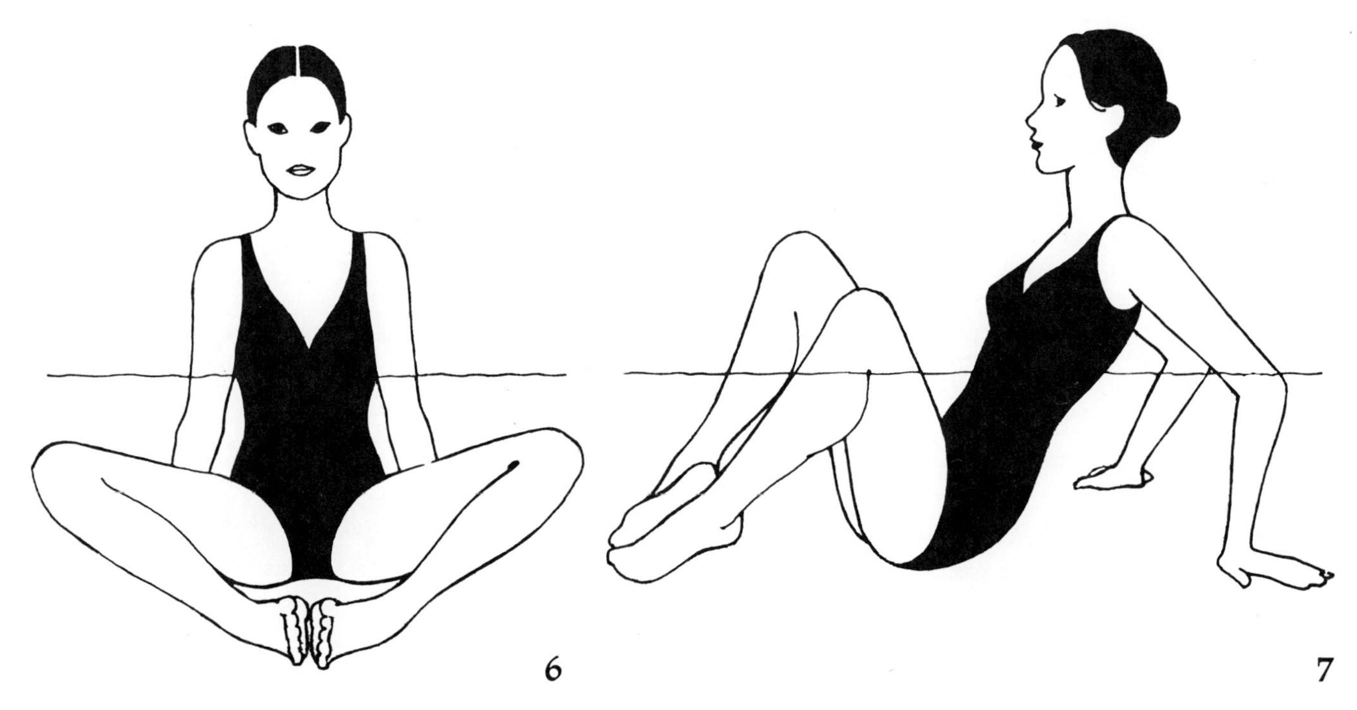

6

7

THE JACK-KNIFE

Further work can be done on the inside of the thighs by taking position **8** where the soles of the feet are facing one another, but not touching, and the legs are some two feet apart. Bring your legs up as close to your tummy as possible against the water pressure, then push them back out to the starting position.

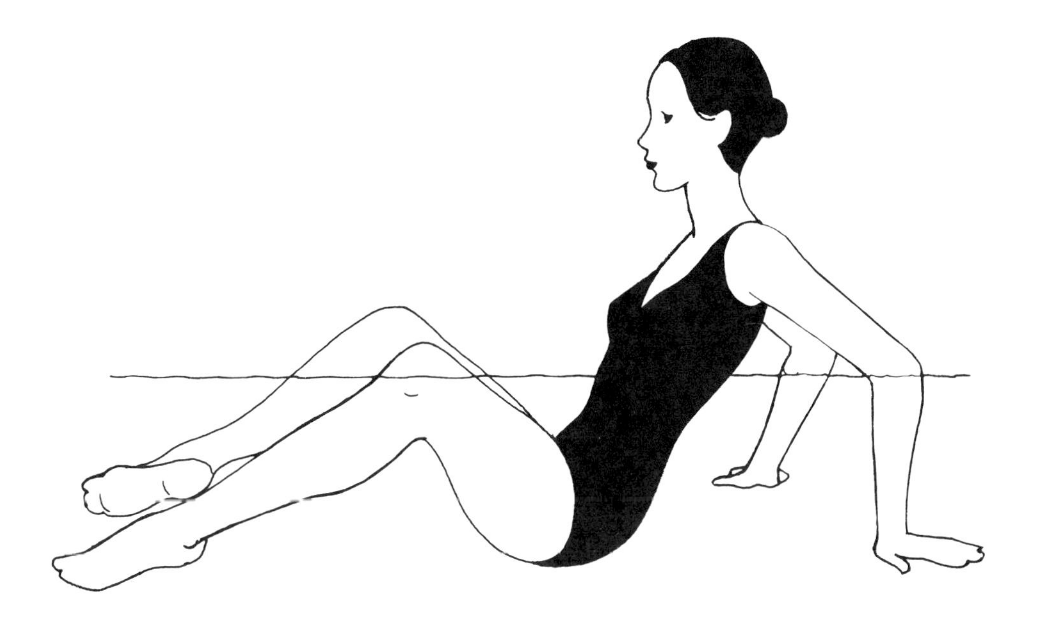

8

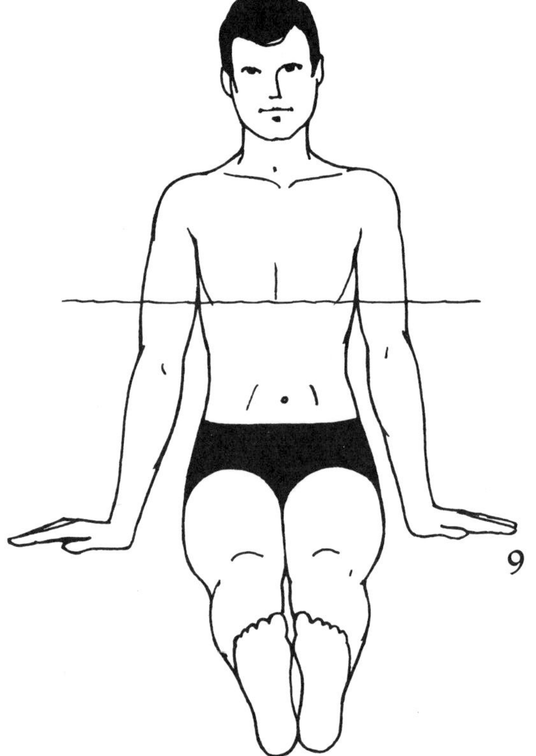

THE SCISSORS

A very strong work-out for the inside and outside of the thighs is started in position **9**. Open your legs as far as possible as shown in **10** against the resistance of the water, and then bring them back to the original position.

THE SUNDIAL

A very difficult area to keep in smooth contour is the back of the thighs and for this position **11** is taken. You should be in water not quite deep enough to support all your weight but enough to take some of the weight off your arms. Bend your knees as shown in **12** and then thrust yourself out of

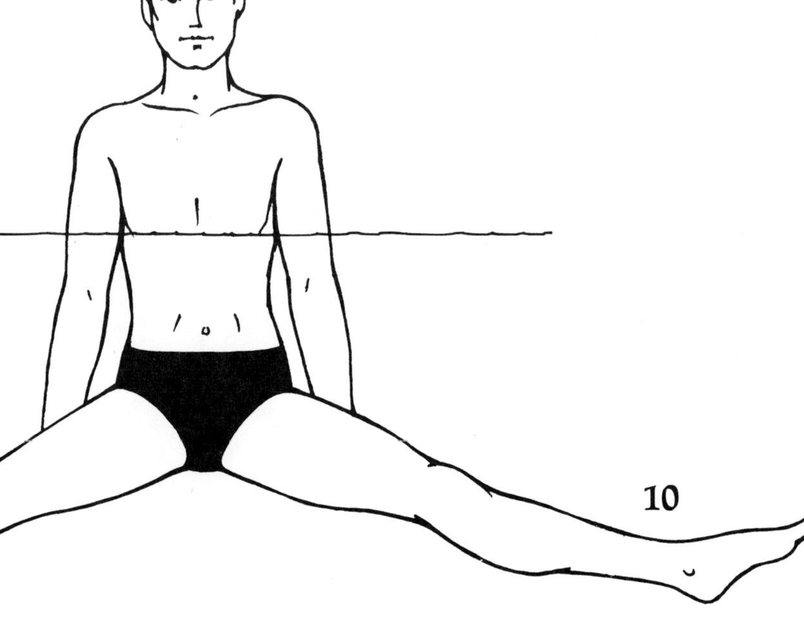

the water. Make sure you have a good bend at the back and your toes are pointing upwards so that the presure of the water is against the soles of your feet. Press them back again.

As in all these exercises, the faster you do the motion the greater the work against the water, but at first do the movements slowly and gracefully until you get a very good form of movement. That is absolutely essential. After a while, when you get stronger, you can learn how to grade the effort on the water pressure.

LEG-LINES

Jumping will strengthen the muscles of the leg but often the jarring contact as you fall back to the surface is too much for ankles that have become weak through months of neglect and little exercise.

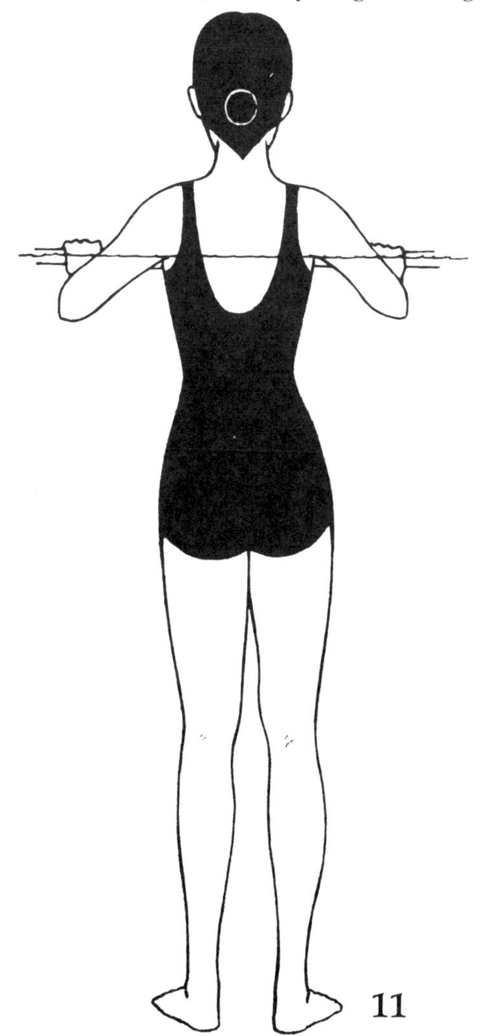

11

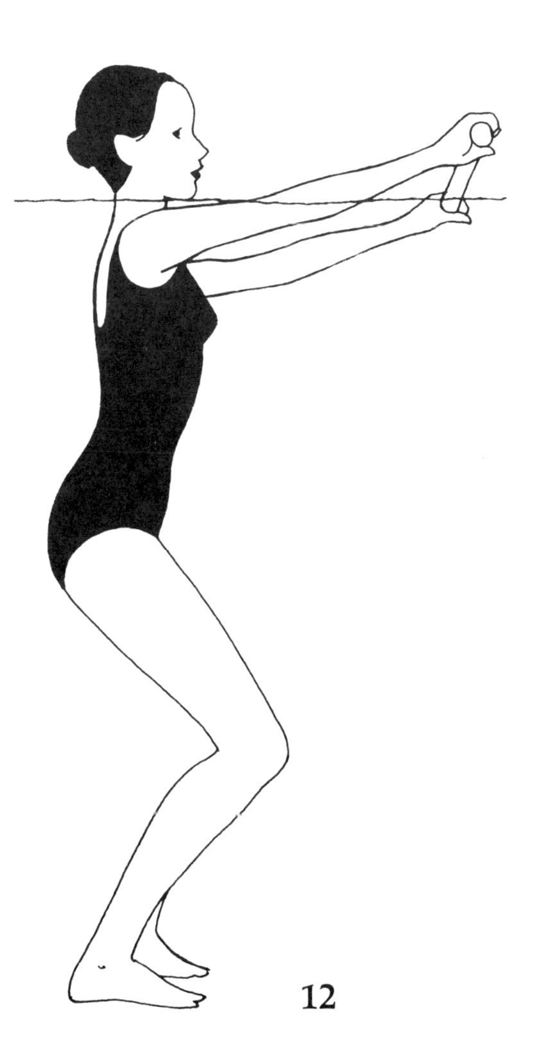

12

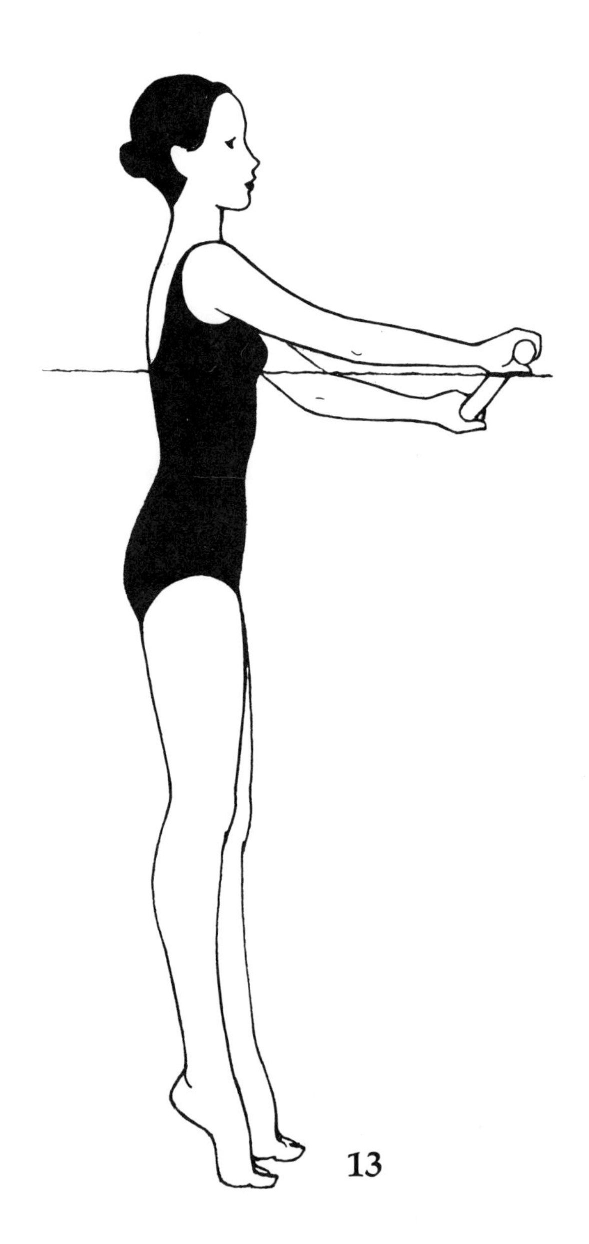

13

JACK-IN-THE-BOX

This exercise strengthens the whole leg but, by reducing the weight of the body by using water to support yourself, the smoothness of the muscle is worked on, so giving a good line to the leg. Here, you start in the swimming-pool by standing with the water just under the armpits and holding on to the bar, as shown in **13.** Gradually bend down a little, and then with a quick thrust, push yourself as high as you can go. As you come down, kick open your legs behind you, as in **14.** Repeat this several times.

The sequence we have just described can also be carried out in the sea or in a swimming-pool without the benefit of a side bar by having a companion hold your arms by his or her hands, or you can put your hands on his shoulders for support.

To get over-all shape of the legs, you have to exercise all the muscles, particularly those on the inside of the leg and at the back of the knee where fat often collects.

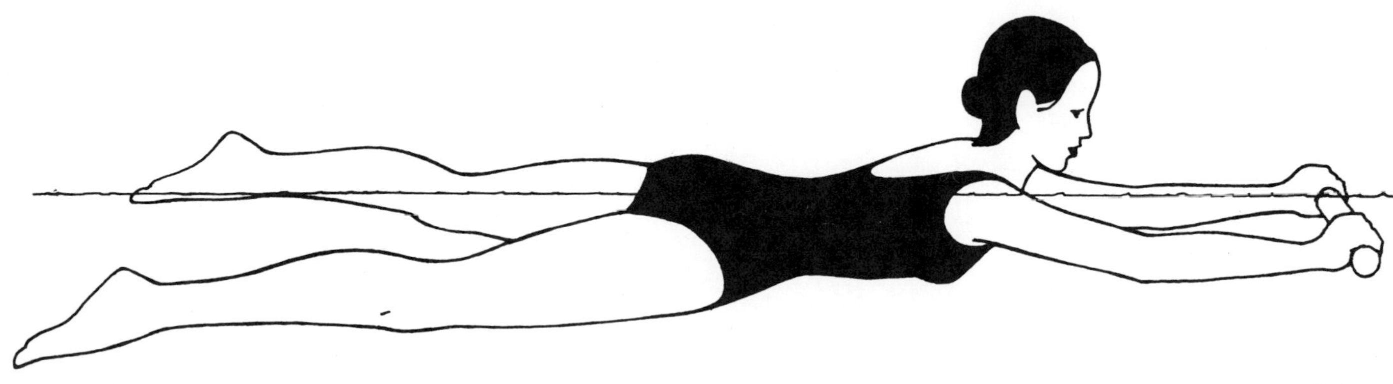

14

The Buttocks

THE PORPOISE

This sequence exercises the large muscles of the buttocks. Take up a position on the bar of the swimming-pool **15,** or have somebody hold you by the hands, or you can hold their arms in the sea, then lie flat out. Now move as if you were doing the breast-stroke, but use only your legs. Do one motion of the breast-stroke of the legs, then, still keeping your legs apart, alternately shape your legs as shown in **16,** first one leg in the air then the other, using very careful, graceful motions all the time. After doing this several times, you then use the crawl motion of the feet, and then go back to **15.** Continue this until you feel quite tired, in which case you can just lie flat on the water. Resistance is increased by the speed with which you do the exercise.

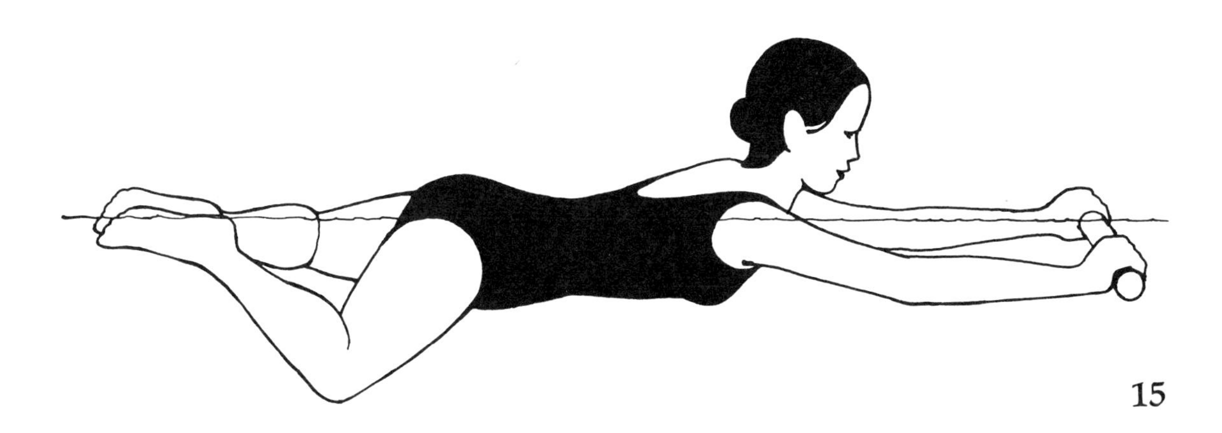

15

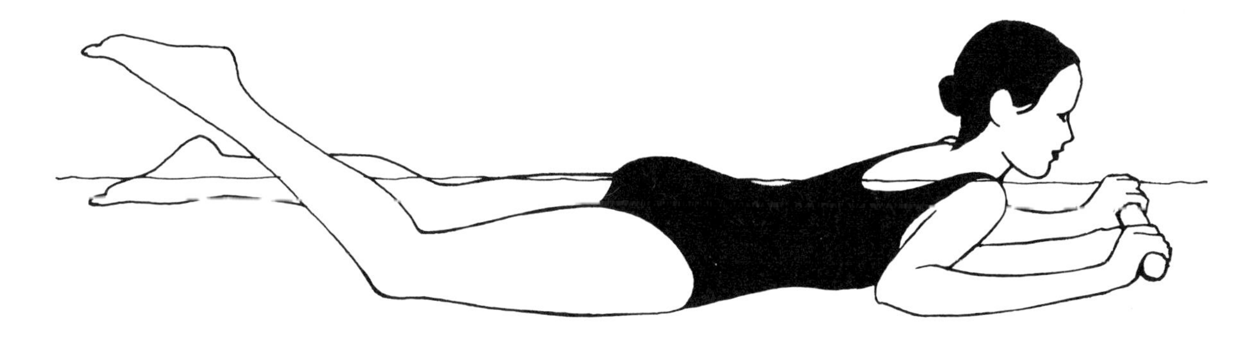

16

THE AQUA DANCE

The sequence that follows, which I call 'aqua dance', really is a very useful exercise for over-all body shaping. It is particularly good for the legs, especially the thighs, and also, because of the resistance to water and the balancing you have to do, it is excellent for co-ordination, posture and the line of the waist. First of all, you need to start with water up to your waistline, but if you find this too difficult try it in much shallower water. Take up position **17**, and then by putting your weight on the right leg, bring up your left leg

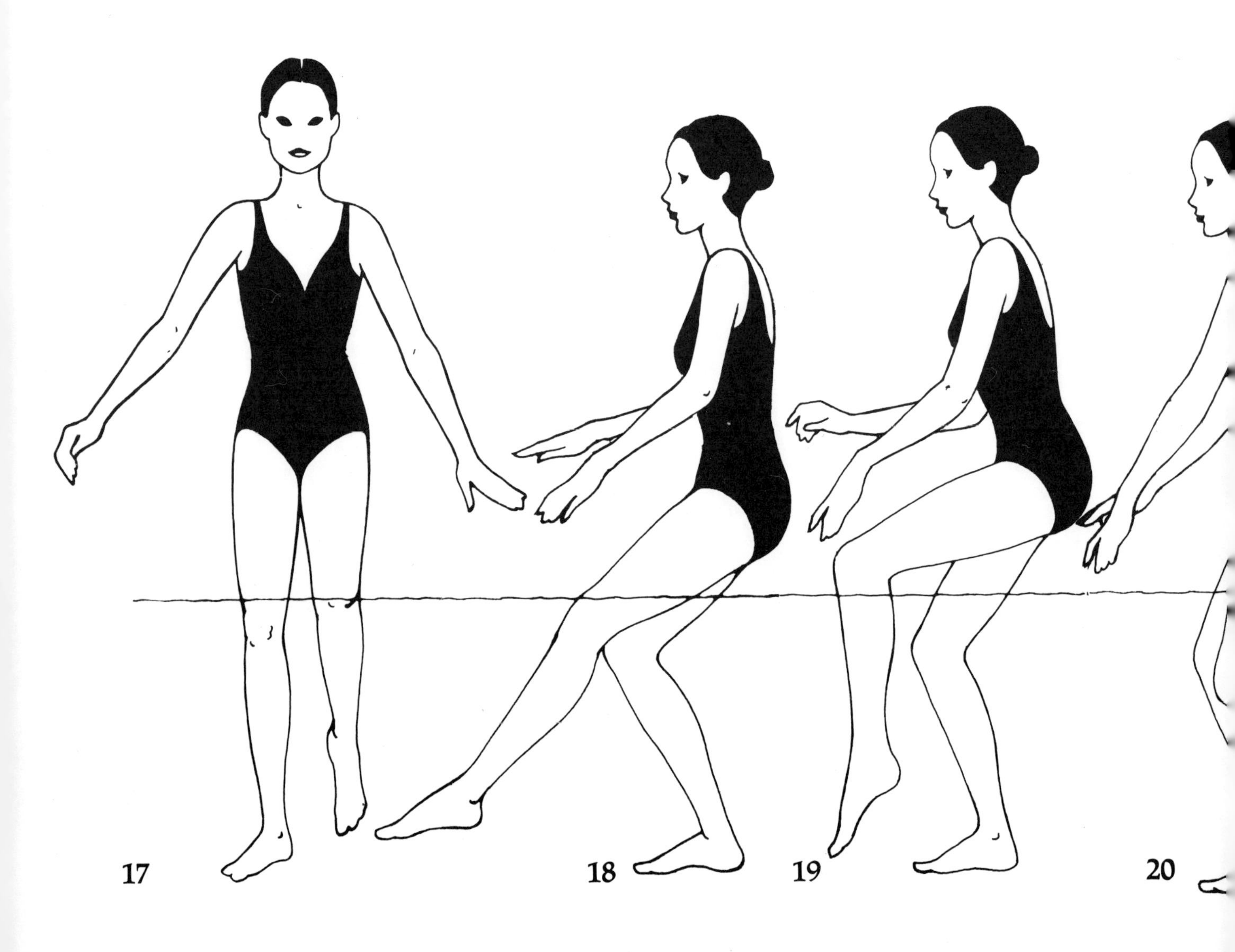

as shown in **18**, pushing against the water and then bring it back as shown in **19**, pushing the sole of your foot against the water as you cross over your leg behind you, right up to position **20**. Change the weight of your body on to your left foot and then bring up your right foot as shown in **21**, which you will notice is a different movement from the one you have just carried out. Push the foot up, then bring it down and across as shown in **22** and bring it back down through **23** to the starting position. Start the whole process again, beginning this time of course with the right leg.

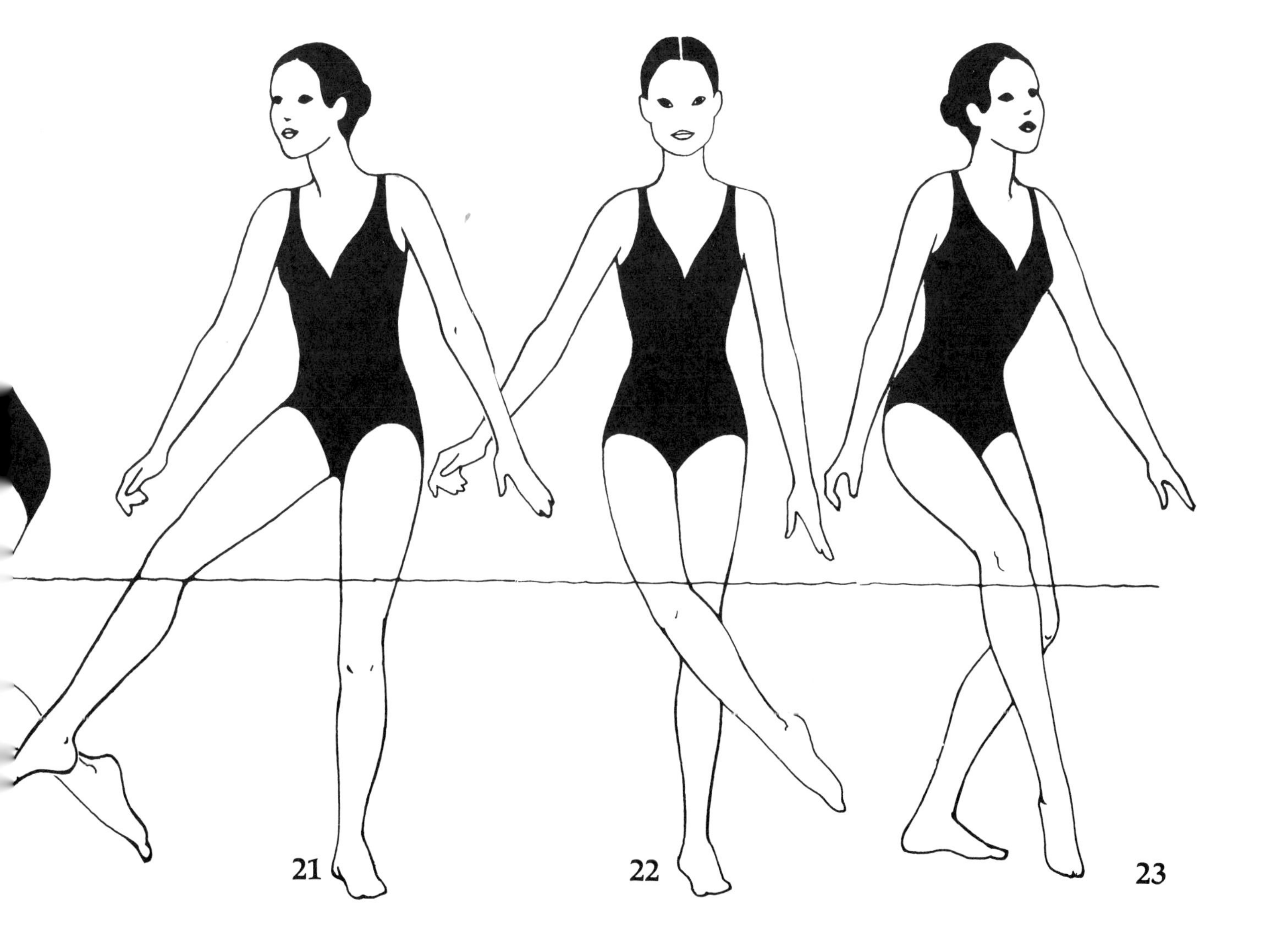

This 'aqua dance' is difficult at first, particularly in water that is more than about a foot deep, but you can grade the work on your leg muscles by first increasing the *speed* at which you do the exercise, and second by the depth of the water. For ordinary shaping purposes you need to have a smooth, flowing motion, but if you need to slim, use water that is about 1 foot deep and do it as quickly as possible.

Regarding the amount of time taken to perform these exercises, it will take a little while to learn to do them well but once you know them thoroughly, the whole sequence should take about 7 minutes. At first just try to do them properly, and then you can build up your repertoire. If you are keen on getting a really good shape, you should work hard enough on them to feel a definite touch of fatigue in the muscles. Once this happens, move on to the next exercise which will use a different set of muscles and so on as you work your way through the whole sequence in this chapter.

These sequences, with about a minute spent on each main exercise, and about 4 minutes spent on the 'aqua dance' every day, are excellent for acquiring and maintaining healthy, beautiful legs.

Chapter Six

WAIST AND HIPS

WAIST AND HIPS

The Waist

A woman's waist is really a wonderful set of shapes, never flat, but curved, dipped, rounded. The shape is made by muscles providing a blue-print of beauty, sealed by springy skin: you cannot be lovely without some fat, because it helps to make the skin smooth and even, but with too much fat you lose the blueprint. Balance counts. Get your muscles toned, and your figure worries are over.

The shape of the waist really depends on muscles. If you slide your finger across your body just above the hip joint, you will feel strong muscles if you press. These sheaths of very powerful muscle groups keep all the inner organs of the abdomen in place. These muscles are reinforced by extremely powerful sheaths of ligaments.

Even if you are not overweight, the muscles and ligaments I have just mentioned may be slack and toneless, and the internal weight of the organs of the abdomen will mean that your tummy will protrude, and form an unattractive shape. This can be evident even in quite thin people. If they are weak, there is a tell-tale bulge beneath the navel and just above the pubic hair, instead of there being a pleasantly curved midriff.

If your muscles are in good tone, they will be, even when relaxed, to a certain extent, in tension. This is what is meant by good tone: a condition that means the shape of the body will be good. This is always seen in very active women who haven't abused their figures.

TUM ONE

For the first exercise, 'Tum one', float on your back with your feet about eighteen inches apart and with your arms outstretched. Draw in your tummy muscles, count to ten, then let them out; count to five, draw them in, count to ten. Repeat this until the muscles begin to feel a little uncomfortable and then stop. It is unwise to do this exercise after you have just eaten.

TUM TWO

To do this exercise kneel down in shallow water with your knees about eighteen inches apart. Look up and draw in the stomach as far as you can so that you are almost touching the backbone, so to speak, with the muscles of your tummy, and do the same counting sequence as before: draw in, hold for a count of ten, let out, hold for a count of five, draw in and so on. Do this until you get tired. The point about these two tum exercises is that you can do them no matter how flabby or overweight you are and they may stimulate you to take a greater interest in physical exercise. But I think you will gain even greater benefit from them if you enlist the help of a friend who can carry out some dynamic work on this section of the body.

TUM DRUMMING

Lie on your back in water, either in the bath or the sea, or float in a swimming-pool, and get you friend to do *gentle* karate chops in quick succession with both hands, up and down an imaginary line from the top of the

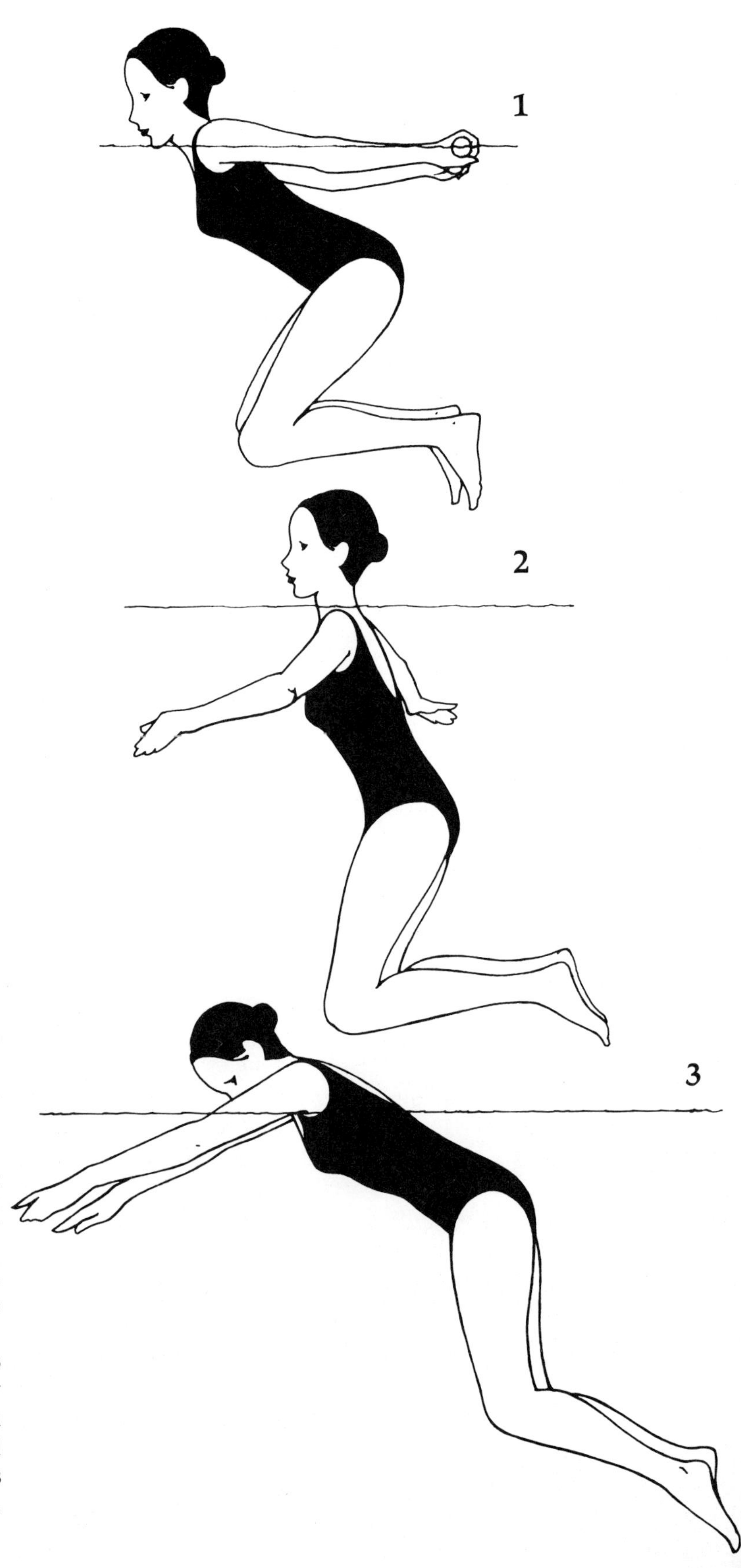

pubic hairs up to the beginning of the rib-cage. Make sure these are not really hard karate chops. They should just go up and down in quick succession, hard enough to make you want to tense your muscles against the impact. Then try 'tum drumming' your partner. When you and your friend become more expert at 'tum drumming', you can start to do the drumming on the area away from this imaginary central line where the waist is. If you do this for five minutes on the midline and five minutes on each side, you will find that the tone of your muscles will improve tremendously. It may also help to dissipate some of the flab that has collected in this region. You should feel around first before drumming to make sure you *never drum the bones.*

To help you in working on this particular area of the body, it is wise to remember that if you distend the stomach—I mean by that the actual stomach inside your body and the intestines—by eating a large amount of food in a very short time, this will militate against a firm midriff. To repeat advice given earlier, you should endeavour to keep the amounts of your meals small and try to eat a greater number of tiny meals rather than two large meals during the day. Similar remarks apply to the drinking of large quantities of liquid. The so-called beer belly, so frequent in men, is, apart from the flab that is over the top of the muscles, also indicative of stretched tendons and ligaments and toneless muscles, which would still appear to give a very bad figure, *even if* the actual flab itself were removed.

Another point which might help you is that women who are sexually *active* rarely suffer from a drooping abdomen. The reason for this is that during intercourse the natural reflexes are allowed to operate, the muscles of the abdomen are naturally contracted,

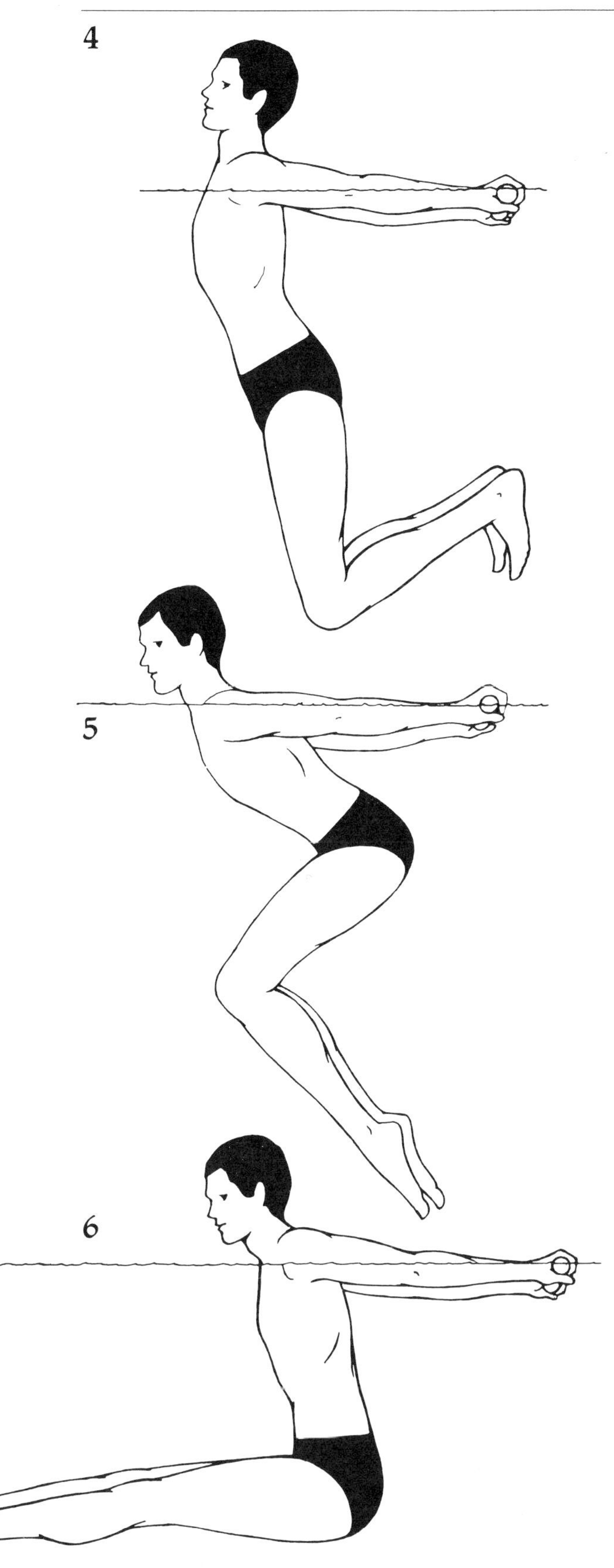

rather like the exercise when you are lying on your back, 'tum one'. It is certainly true to say that sexual enjoyment is improved if you do contract the tummy muscles, particularly those down from the chest to the pubic arch. In frigid women and impotent men, these muscles are very rarely contracted. The belly is protruded outwards. In healthy people the tummy muscles go into waves of contraction and relaxation.

The Hips

If you have a good waist it's very difficult not to have good hips, so the exercises for both tend to be related. The main point to notice is the line from the waist over the hips down on to the thigh. The several different sets of muscles in this area can be exercised together, and this is the object of the following sequences.

KING PENGUIN

Take up position in the swimming-pool in water 4 foot deep or more, holding the bar with the feet against the wall **1**. Let go of the bar, pushing hard with your feet against the wall and diving out, as shown in **2** and **3**. This is quite a dynamic sort of exercise and now you have to go back to the bar. Taking up the position again in **4**, this time push off against the wall but instead of letting go with the hands, hold on tightly and sweep your body round as shown in **5** until you end up in position **6**. Then curl back to the beginning shown in **4**. This exercise is a very powerful strengthener of the front and side of the hip, of the waist and the small of the back.

THE METEOR

Take up position **7** on the bar of the swimming-bath and push yourself off by letting go of the bar but this time your feet are holding on to the bar so that as you sweep backwards through **8, 9** and **10,** you are holding your position on the side of the swimming-bath with your feet. Stretch out as far as you can. Bring your arms round, as in **11**, back to the position from which you started via **12** so that you are again back at 7. It is a good powerful exercise, for the middle body as well as the shoulders. It helps the legs too, because you have to hold yourself by them. Try this exercise with a partner. This time use exactly the same sort of movements with your partner holding your ankles and your hands on his or her shoulders.

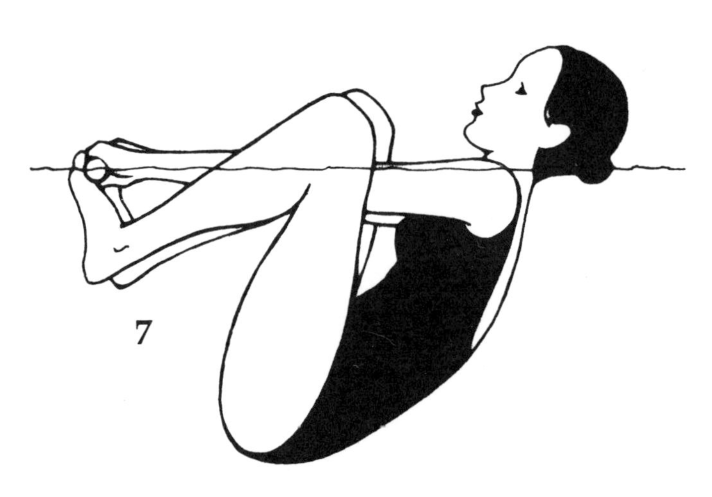

7

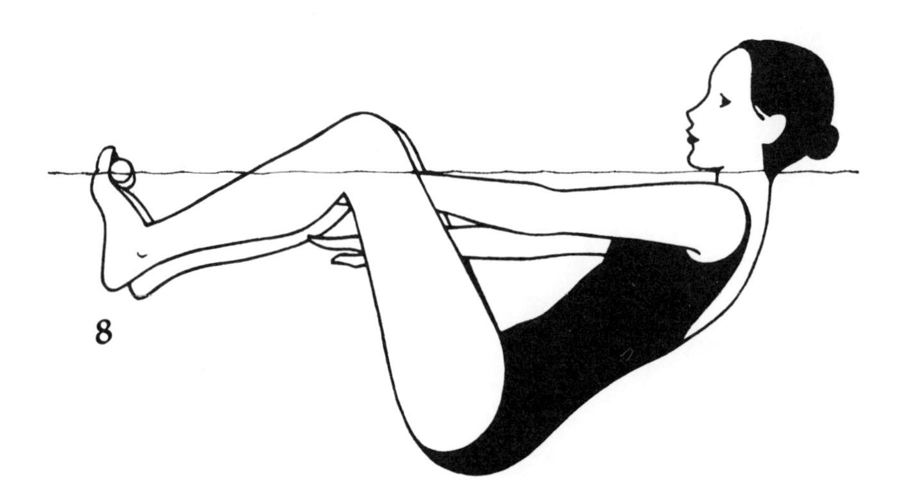

8

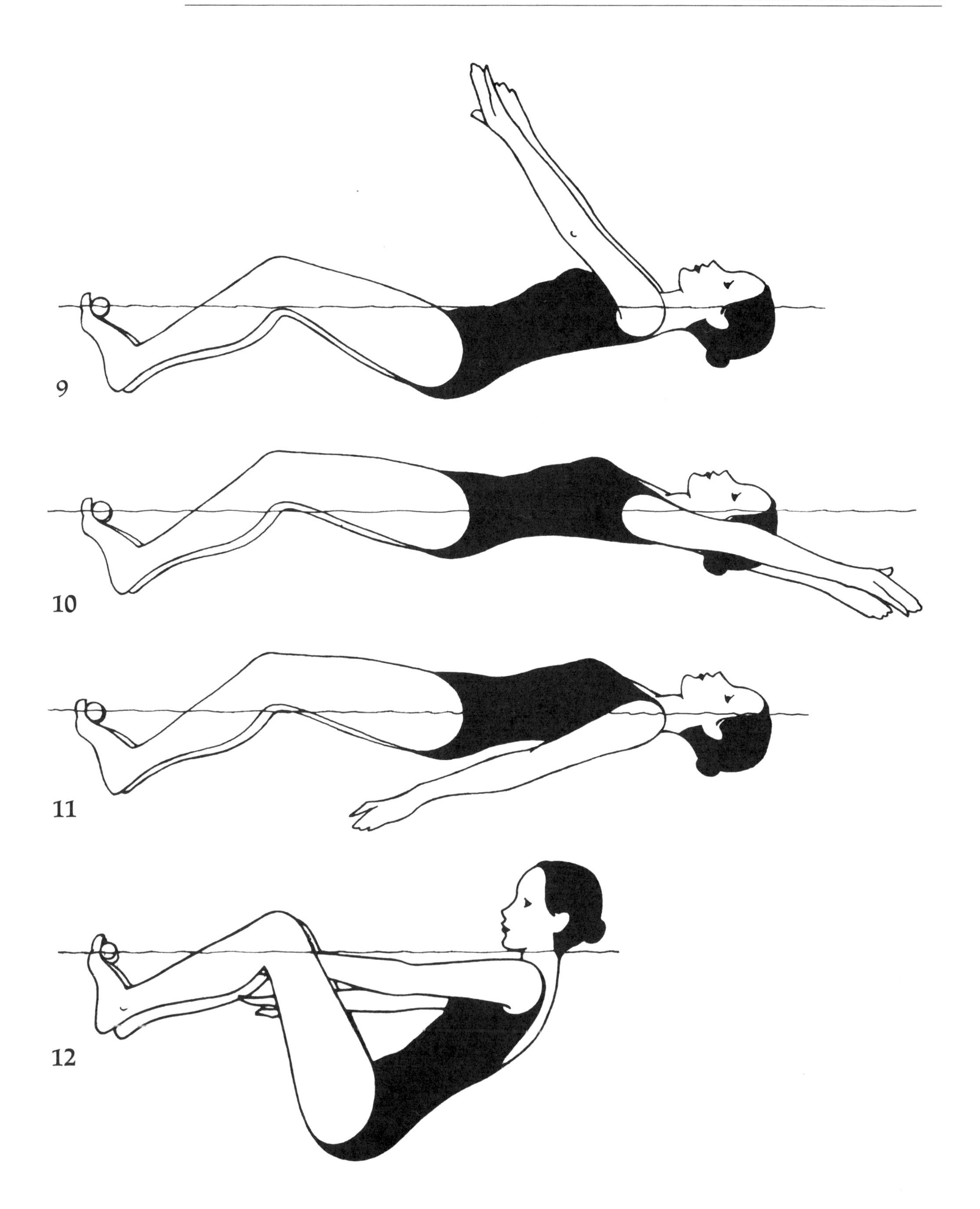
9
10
11
12

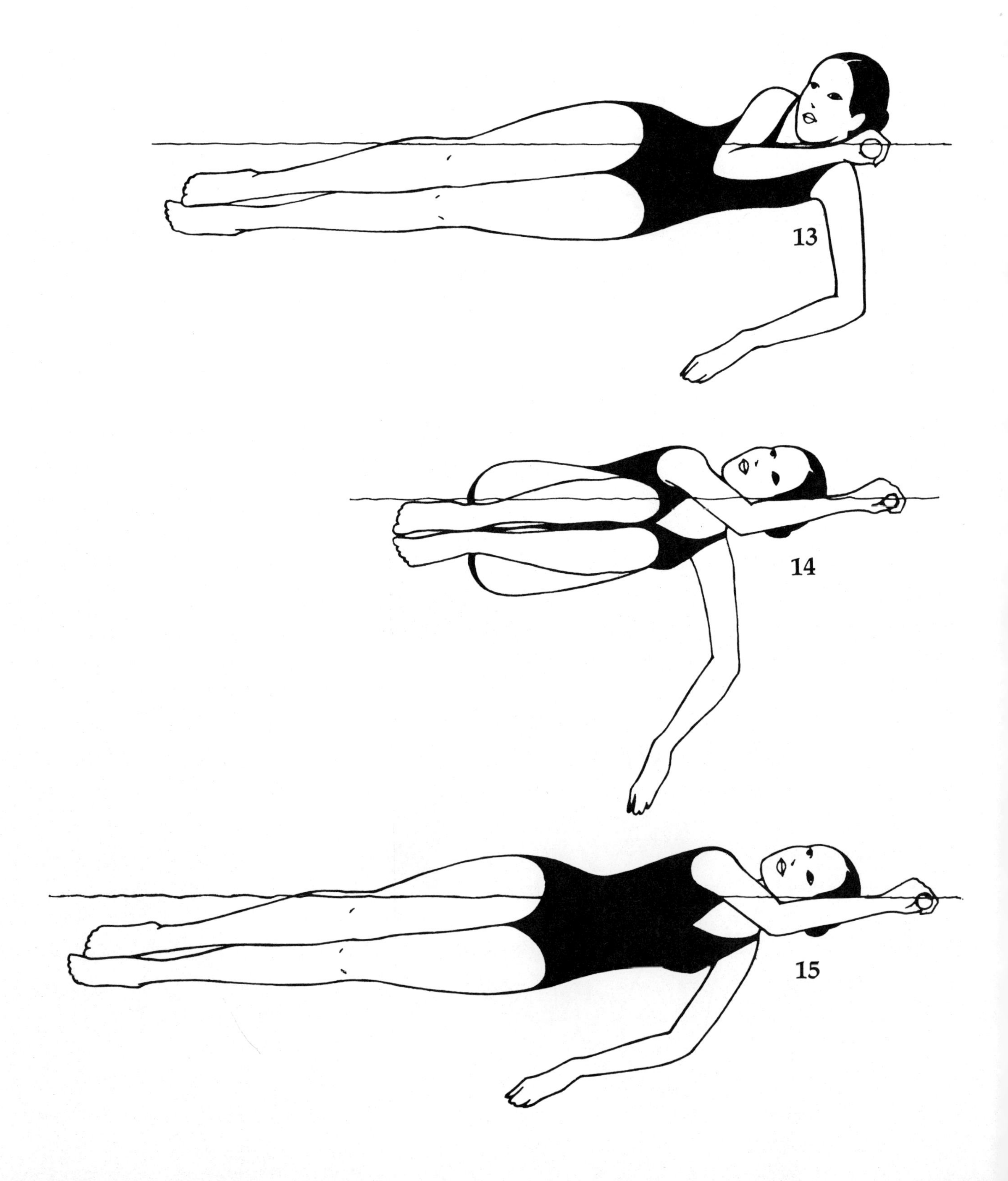
13
14
15

THE MARZIPAN

Another powerful exercise for the whole body, and giving good lines to the tummy and strengthening the arms, begins with position **13**. Hold on to the bar with one hand, with the other one against the wall, so that you are out in a straight line, at right-angles to the side. Bring your thighs up towards your tummy as shown in **14**. Press your legs out to end up in position **15**, then continue bending your legs round as far as you can go as shown in **16**. Sweep them back, pressing your thighs against the water to finish in **17**. Then relax out into the beginning position and start again. After doing this 3 or 4 times change hands and do it exactly the opposite way.

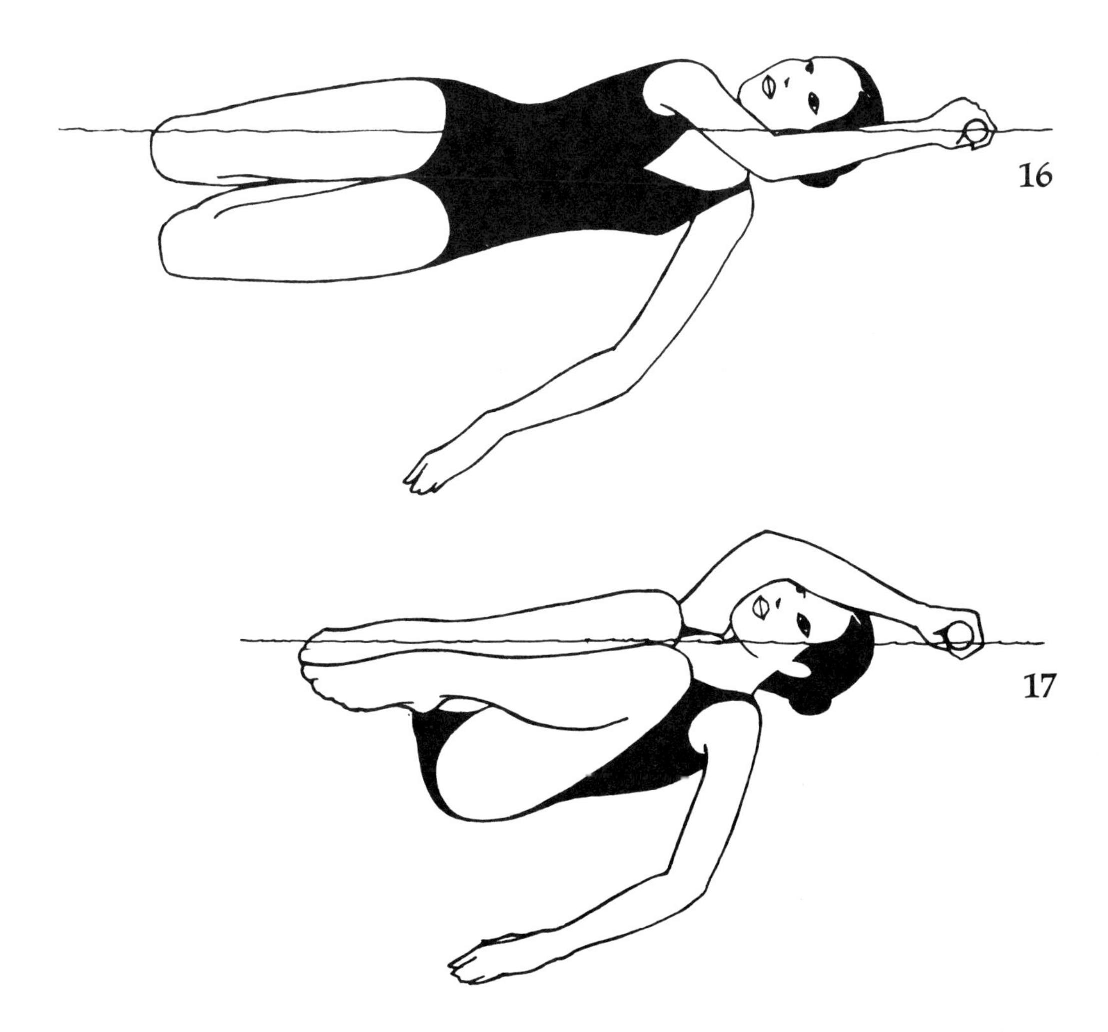

THE CORKSCREW

If you take up position **18** you can exercise your shoulders and your hips and tummy by doing a twirling motion, letting go with your left hand, turning round in the water so that you end up through **19** into **20.** Continue either along the bath, or reverse twirl to where you started from. This can be great fun with a line of partners, if you can get that number of people together.

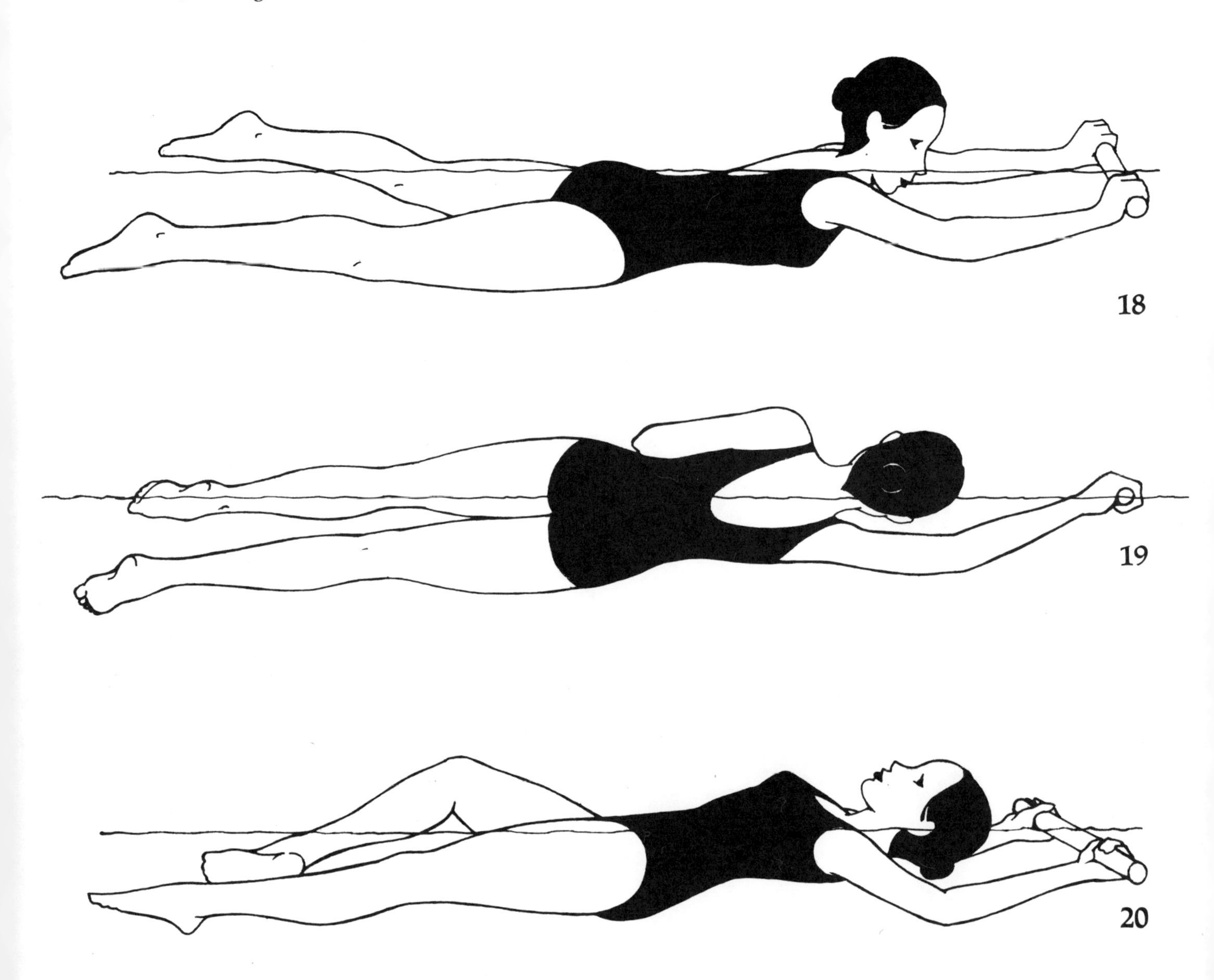

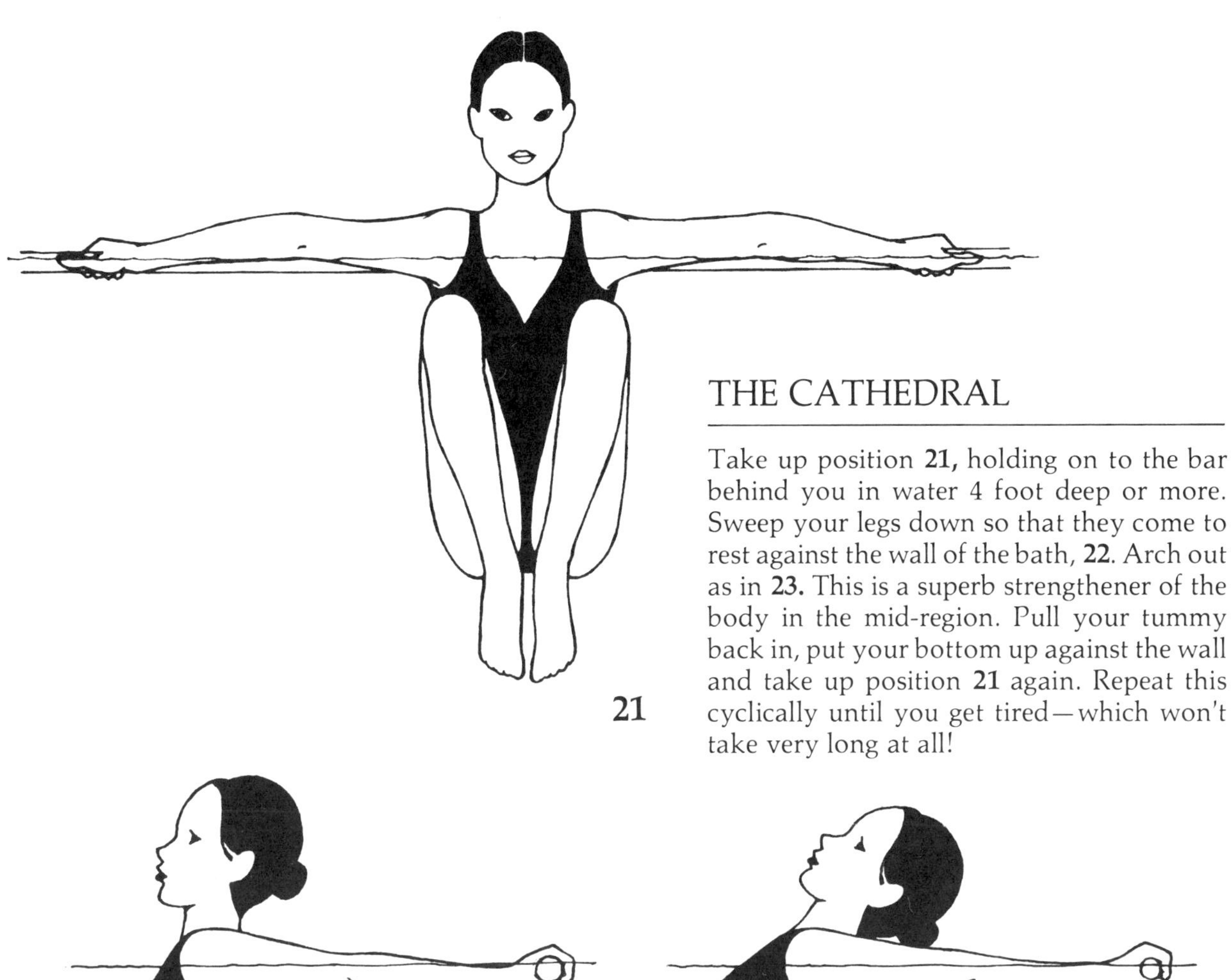

21

THE CATHEDRAL

Take up position **21,** holding on to the bar behind you in water 4 foot deep or more. Sweep your legs down so that they come to rest against the wall of the bath, **22**. Arch out as in **23.** This is a superb strengthener of the body in the mid-region. Pull your tummy back in, put your bottom up against the wall and take up position **21** again. Repeat this cyclically until you get tired—which won't take very long at all!

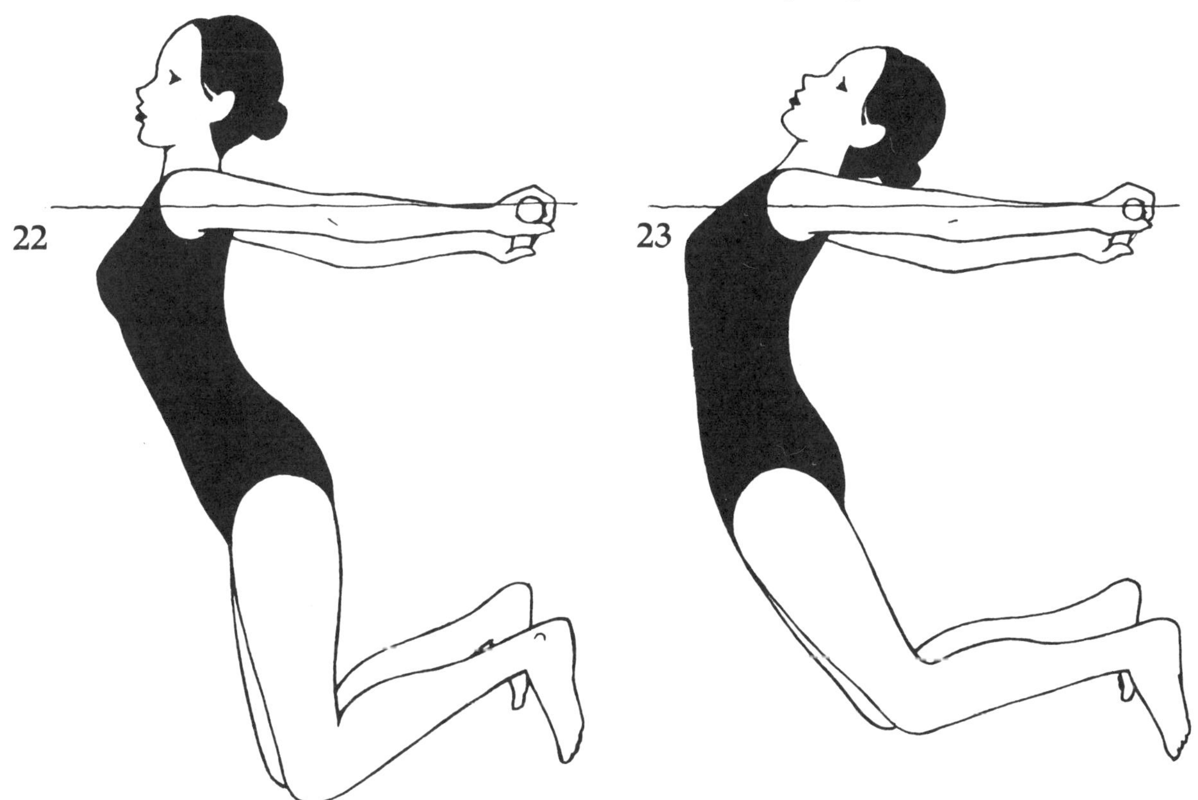

22

23

WATER TWIST

Try this free-standing exercise, shown in **24**, where the water is just about up to your chest (or to the waist at first). Put your hands in the position shown, steady yourself on your feet and swing down as shown in **25** until you get round to the other side as shown in **26**. Sweep your feet back down again by changing the hand position as shown in **27** to end up in **24** again. Do this several times for one side, then the other. You will feel a definite pull on both sides of the waist when doing this. It's also very good for improving the line of the arms and legs.

All these exercises are powerful muscle

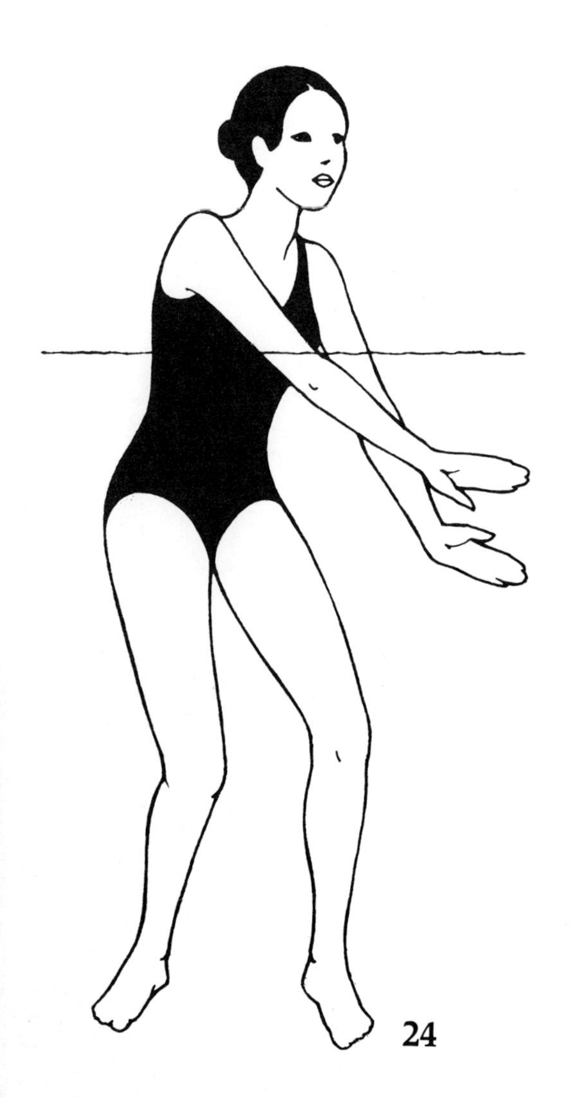

24

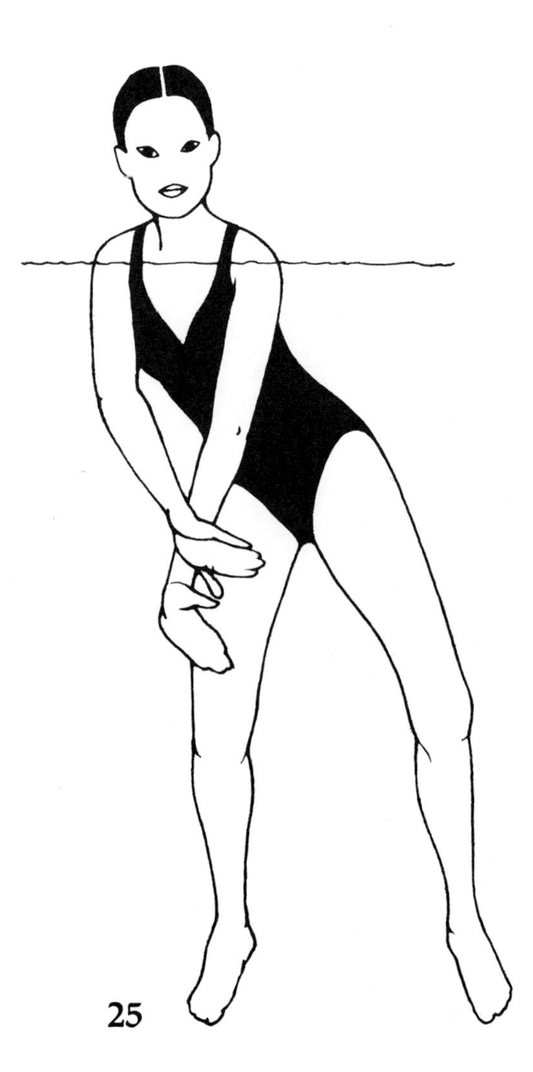

25

builders. If you want to put on weight, you can use the technique in a very much harder fashion. As with usual slimming techniques, you just need to do them a few times each, but if you are a man trying to put on heavy muscle you will have to spend many minutes at this work, working very hard by increasing force on the water until you are tired. After a rest, repeat, then rest. The next day do not do any work on that particular area at all. For ordinary slimming and shaping purposes you need only spend a few minutes having fun doing the exercise until you feel a definite pull in the muscles, at which point you should continue for a few more seconds, then stop.

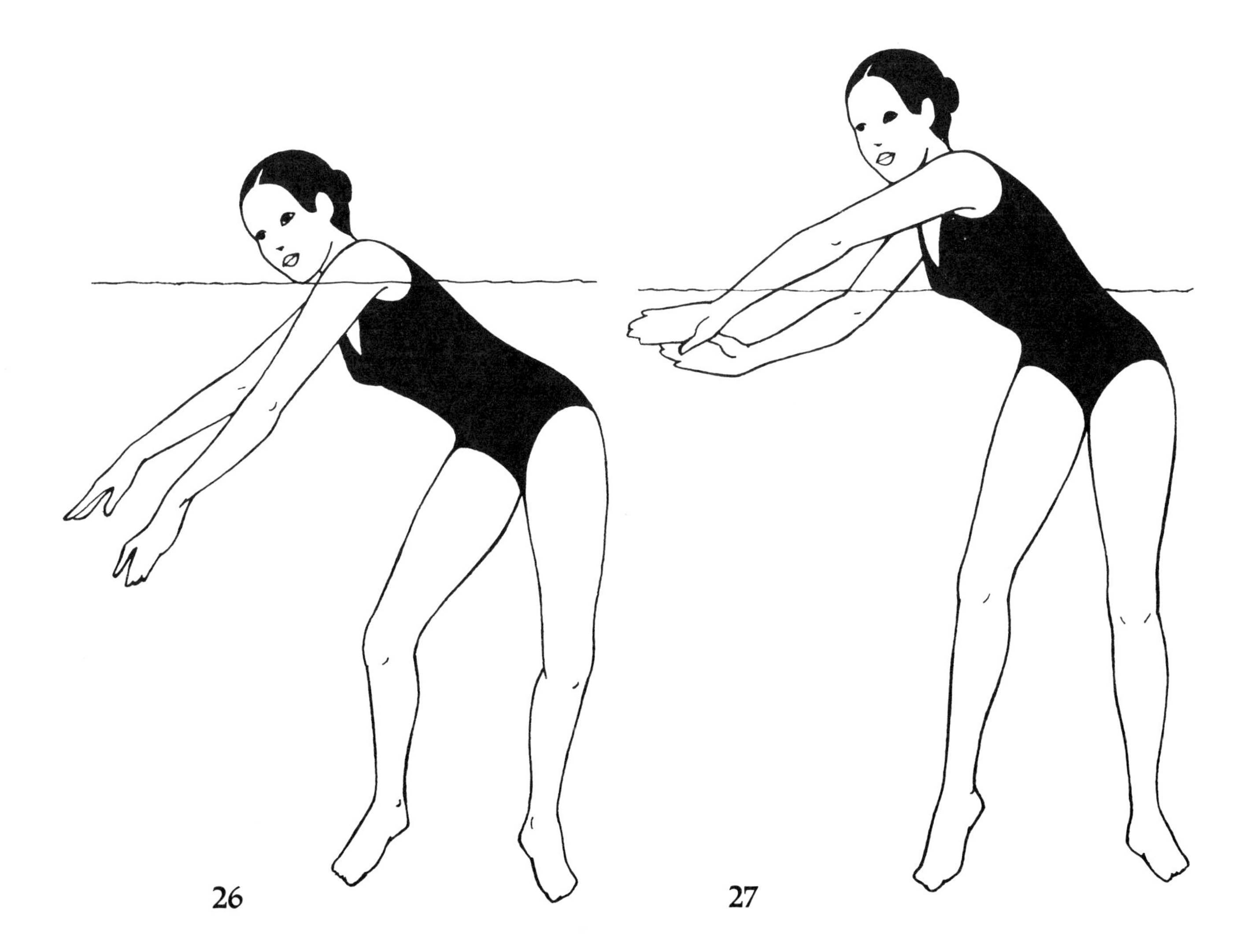

26 **27**

AQUA TWIST

In this exercise, hold on to the bar in the deeper end of the swimming-pool so that you are floating on the water. Bend your knees up as shown in **28** and then do a sort of twisting dance as shown in **29** and **30.** If you find this too difficult—it does take a considerable amount of co-ordination—try the easier form starting at **31** with the feet on the swimming-pool floor, using exactly the same motion, switching from side to side. This exercise will give you a good line on the outside of the waist, over the hips and down on to the thighs. If you do this to music it is great fun. A total sequence is **31, 32** to **33** to **34**.

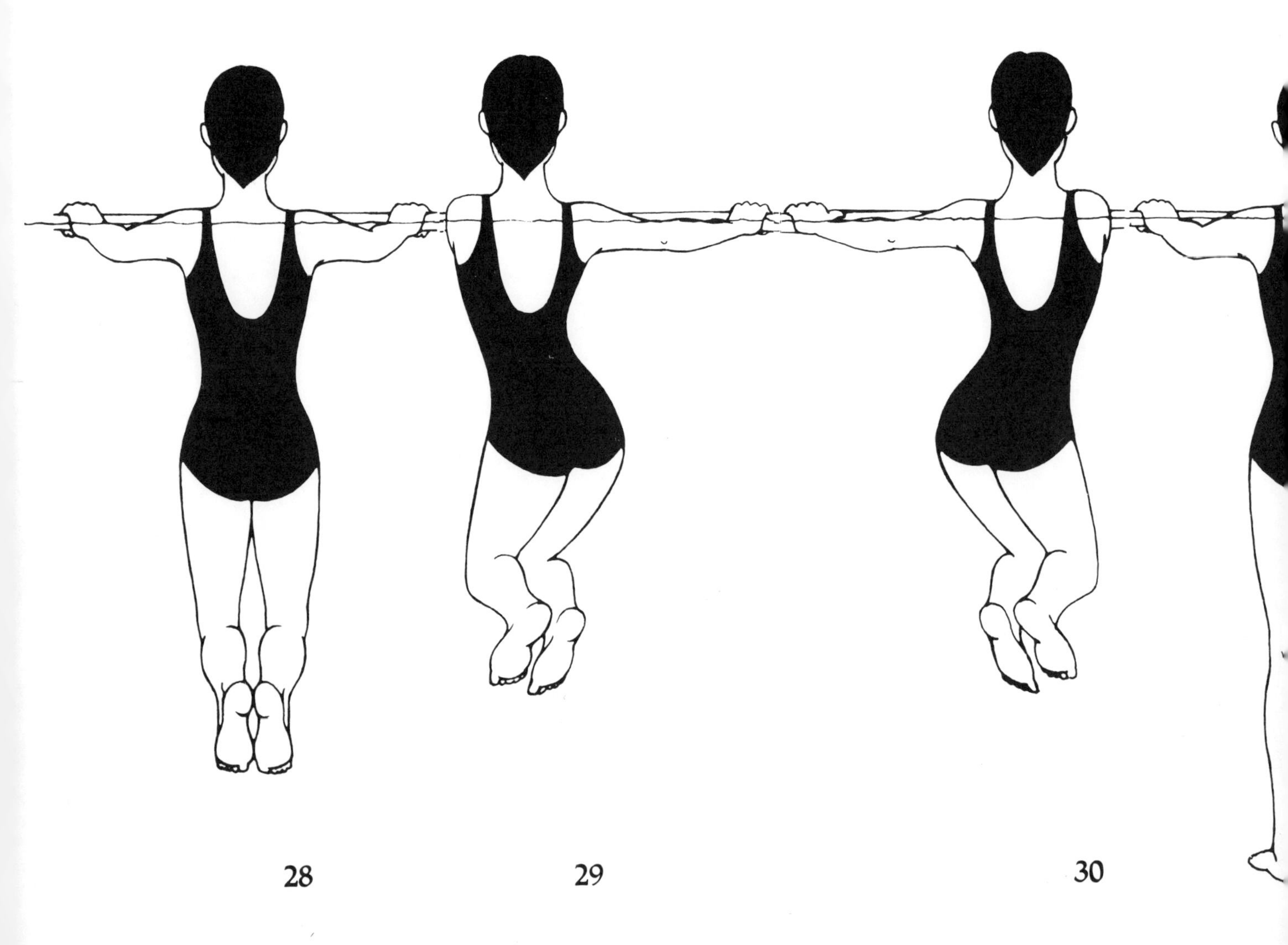

28 29 30

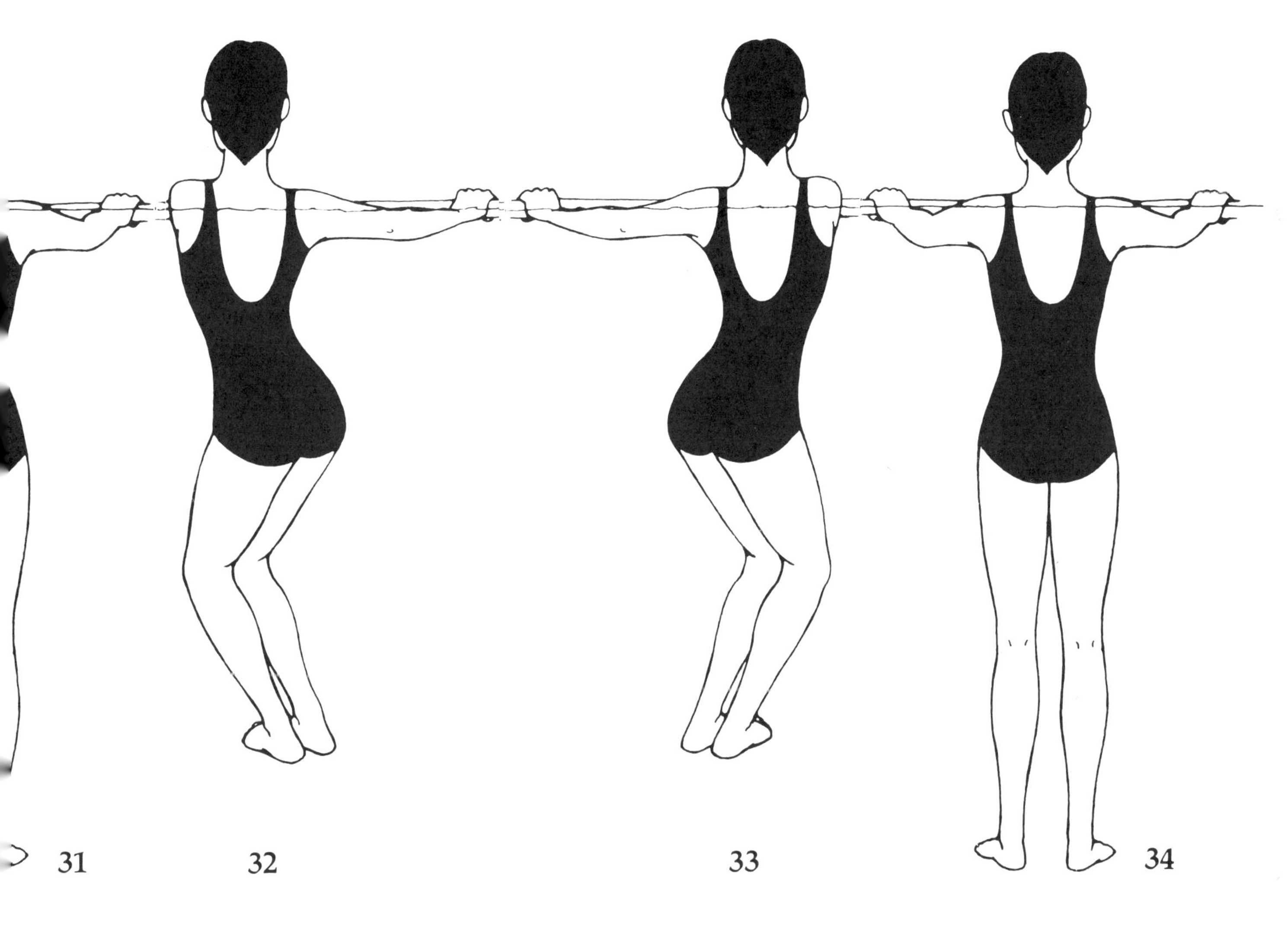

31 32 33 34

HORIZON TWIST

Again working on the mid-part of the body, take up position **35** lying flat out on the water, draw up your legs slightly and twist to one side as shown in **36** then twist right around to the opposite side as shown in **37,** holding firmly on to the bar. Repeat until you feel just a little fatigued.

Vary this work by then taking up position **38**, lying flat out in the water holding tightly on to the bar behind you. Twist as shown in **39** through **40** to **41** and keep the motion up until you feel a definite pull in the muscles.

These twisting exercises from **35** up to **41** can all be done with someone holding your hands in the sea, or in the swimming-pool if you don't have a bar to work against.

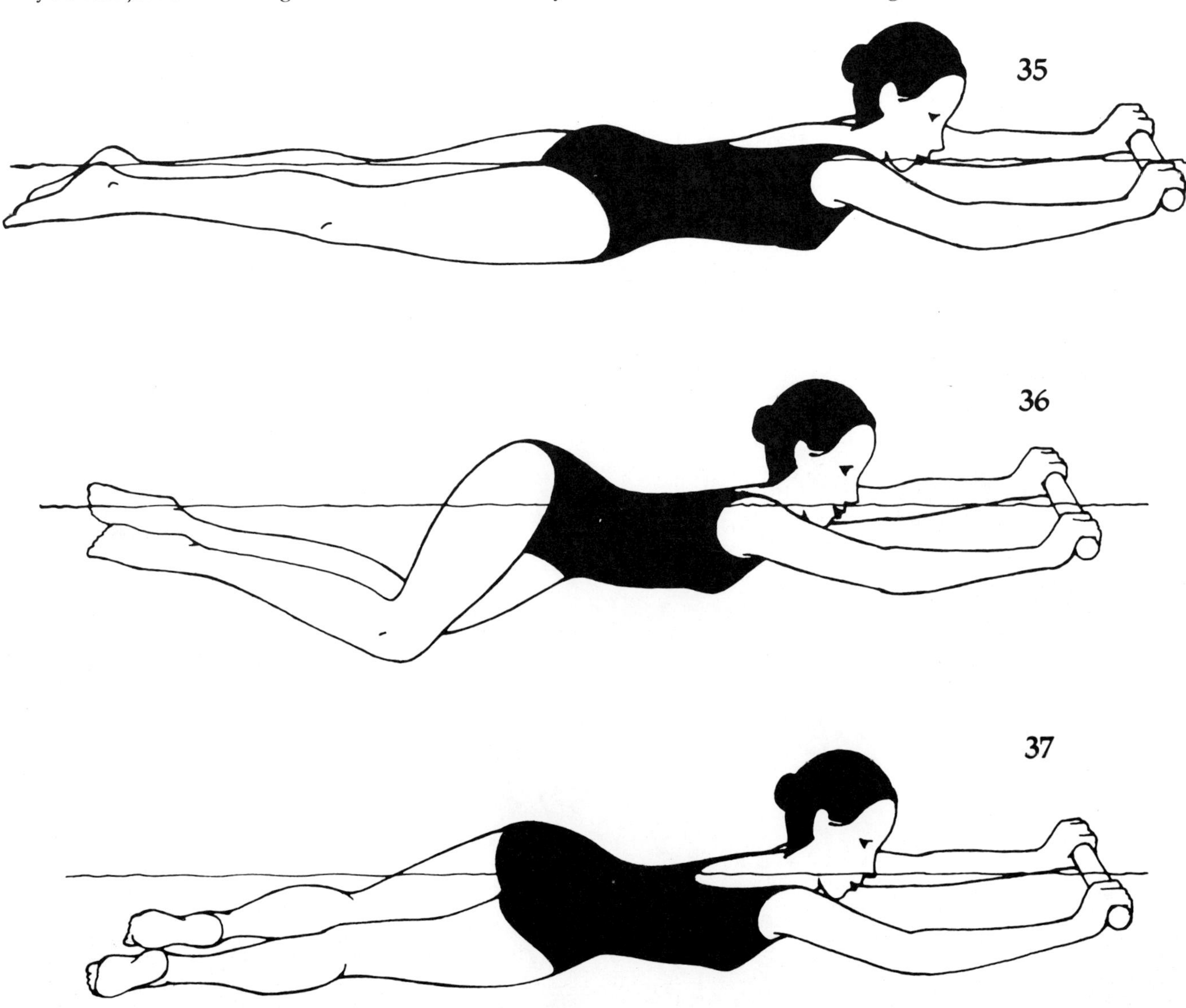

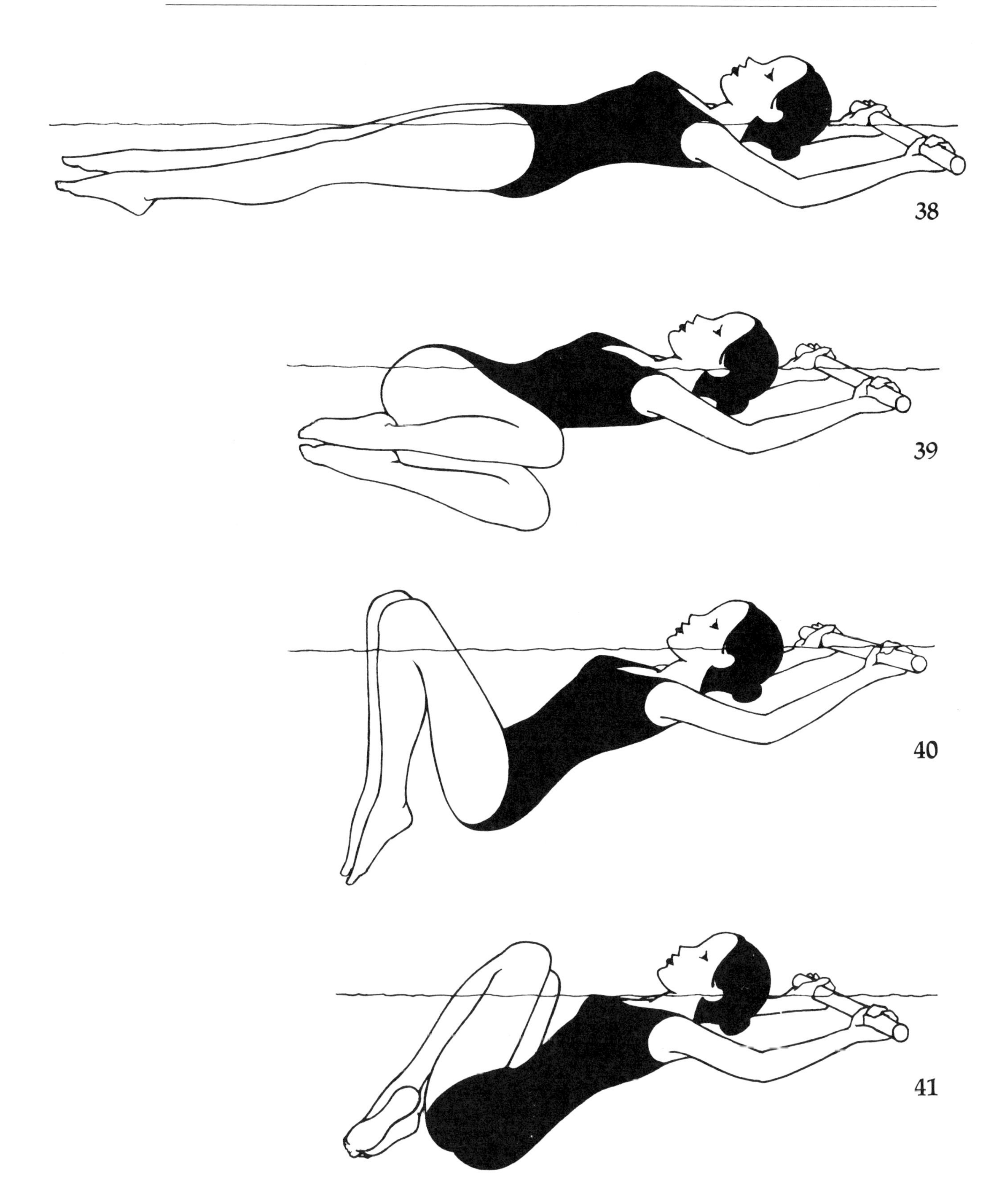
38
39
40
41

THE JET

To finish off try this explosive type of exercise. It takes the weight, so to speak, off the muscles of the tummy which you've been working on and improves the line that we are discussing: the line of the thighs, up on to the hips and up to the waist. Take up position **42.** At first you can use quite shallow water but in time you go below the surface. Force yourself up on your feet, putting your hands up like a diver going upwards (rather than down) as shown in **43,** bringing them up into position **44** and then you are off, **45**. You should be able to raise yourself several feet out of the water by this technique.

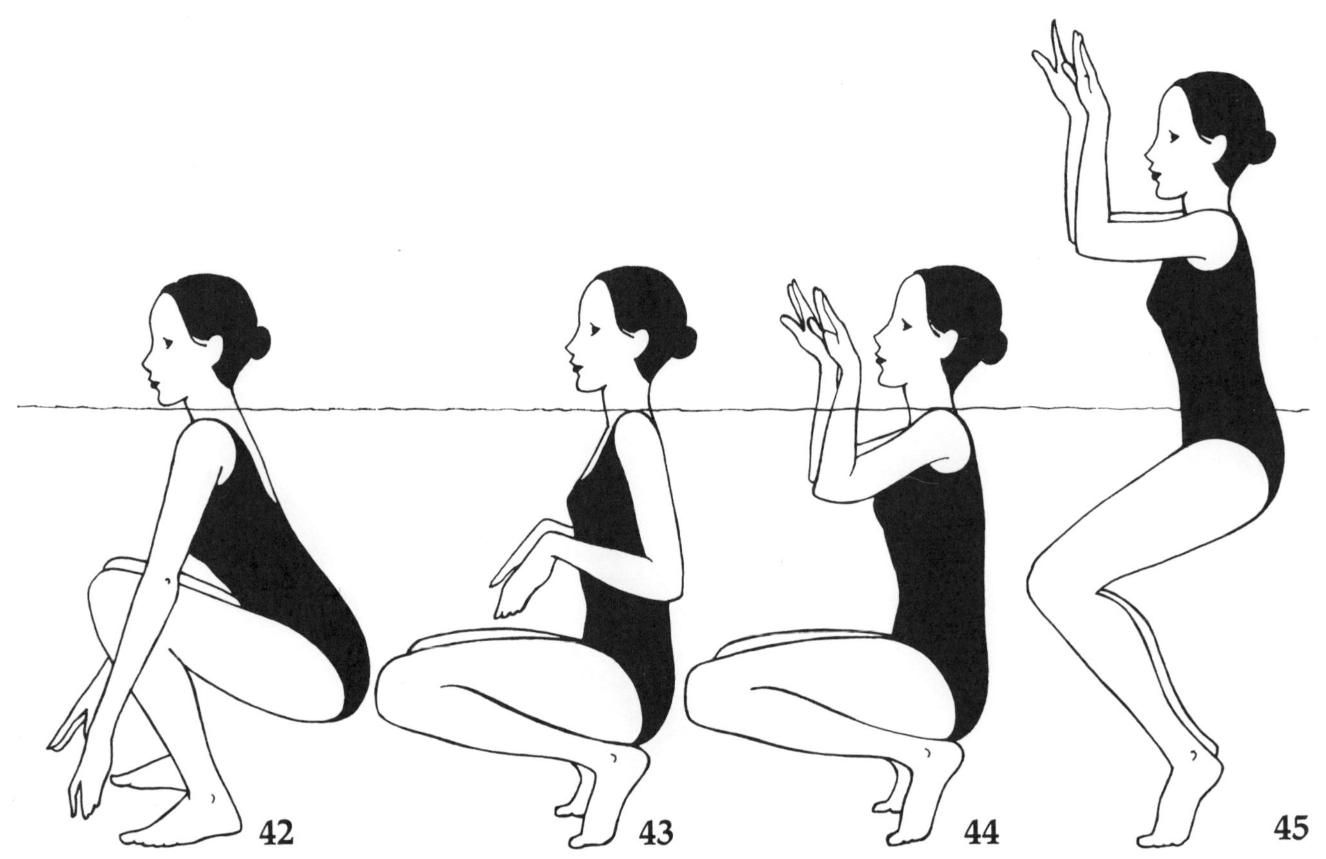

Chapter Seven

THE UPPER BODY

THE UPPER BODY

Our arms are capable of a great number of different movements. The shoulders can make full circular movements, and the elbow and wrist, although more restricted, can also make many actions. Unfortunately, we do not use all this potential in our everyday life, because we perform jobs which require only limited action. Often when we change our jobs, or suddenly use these neglected movements, we pull our tendons and strain our muscles, simply because they haven't been kept in good tone.

From the point of view of beauty, full movements are essential, because only in that way will all the muscles be exercised, and assume their normal fullness, to give a good line to the arm, particularly at the upper arm, and at the shoulder. By exercise, the flow of blood is improved, and this helps to prevent fat from building up, while during weight reduction the blood takes the liberated fat from under the skin to other parts of the body to be burned as fuel for energetic movements, and the waste is expelled in our normal breathing-out process.

People who do not exercise their bodies soon become stiff and incapable of sudden movements without hurting themselves. This fact has led to the belief that after thirty you are 'past it', whereas you should have another forty years of very active life ahead of you. My exercises here can help keep joints and muscles supple, stave off the effects of neglect, improve line and performance. You will soon see, when you do the exercises, how they use your arms and shoulders, wrists and hands, in ways neglected for many months, or even for years. These exercises are also excellent for very young people, who need a balanced development rather than one that is one-sided and which is often the result of the indiscriminate playing of popular or compulsory games.

The upper part of the body also includes the back, the chest and the upper part of the waist, so here, too, I have given exercises to strengthen and exercise these parts of the body. The back in particular tends to suffer from too much sitting-down work, while the chest needs to be exercised since it has very large muscles underneath the breast. These exercises stretch the back and lift the chest, which is excellent for a woman's bust line.

Hands

Our hands are very good at stroking, gripping, picking, flicking, slapping; they are very bad at punching and not well designed for pushing. An inactive hand will lose half its strength in a fortnight. A woman's hand is some twenty per cent smaller than a man's, and about half as strong. It can learn elaborate techniques, like those of a concert pianist, or it can be ignored, so that it atrophies. A beautiful hand is an exercised hand.

It is very simple to gauge a person's health by their hands. A clean well looked after but work worn hand is usually strong to touch, warm, of good colour and relaxed. The healthy hand is in a persistent but very minor steady tremor, of about one two hundredth of an inch. This is caused partly by the pulse, but also by the healthy nervous activation of muscles, making them contract, then relax, in the natural pulsation of living tissues.

It is particularly important to strengthen your hands if you use them in your work. It is even more important if you do use your hands for a fixed number of repetitive actions (as for example typing). You will find that the water exercises help keep your hands supple. If you massage them they get very strong.

Wrists and Arms

THE PADDLE STEAMER

Take up position **5** and scoop the water with your hands, as shown. When you get to the end of the movement depicted in **6**, pull back to where you started.

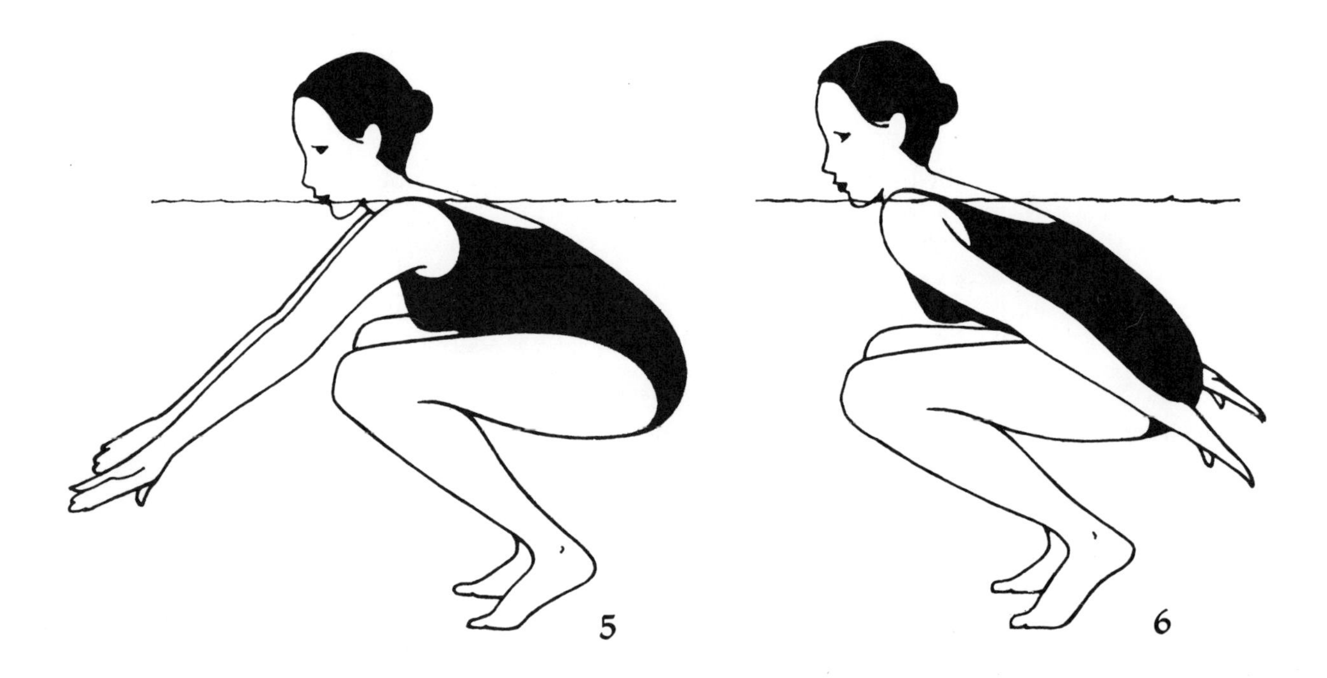

THE CORVAIR

If you assume position **7** and pull the arms out in the wide sweeping motion that you will find in the end position, **8**, you exercise not only the arms but also the chest muscles; that is very good for the bust. You can get a greater pressure by doing the movement very quickly. You can also vary the motion by standing with your palms together so that you exercise the outside of the arm. Another time you can start with palms facing outwards. In other words, you start with the backs of your hands together.

The sequence just described is very good for men who wish to build powerful arms, because the stronger you get, the faster you go through the water, and the faster you go through the water, the more work you do and the more muscles you exercise.

These first two sequences for general shaping should be done approximately 5 times each, with the water level hardly above the elbow. It's harder work, of course, if you go into deeper water.

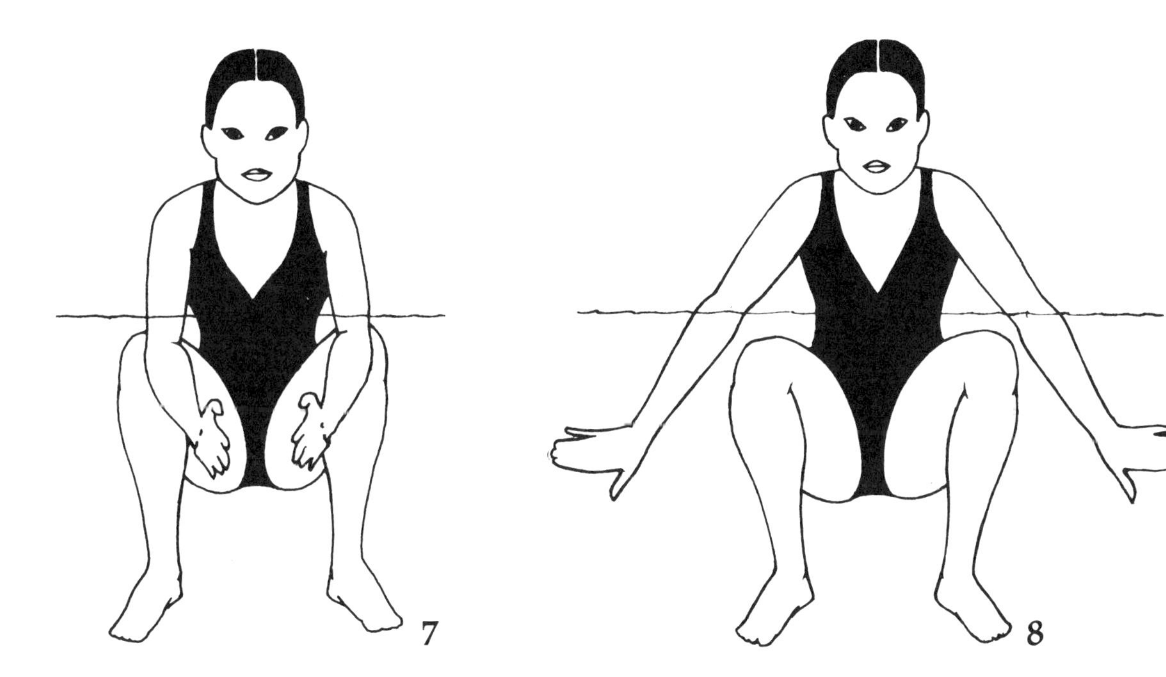

Shoulders

THE GLADIATOR

To develop strong, powerful chest muscles or a good, firm bust line, while exercising the top muscles of the shoulders, take up position **1,** standing in the water, and, with considerable force, come down into the water as shown in **2,** bringing your arms through into **3** then return them to **1.** This exercises the side of the chest and also the muscles upon which your breasts rest. A variation of this exercise which also exercises the tummy muscles is shown in **4** whereby you force down the water with your hands as you go down vertically. Bend you knees and your back. The deeper you go the harder it is. For normal shaping, this sequence can be repeated 4 or 5 times. For slimming, you shouldn't do it too fast or work too hard. For body-building you should go as deeply into the water as you can and work as hard as you can.

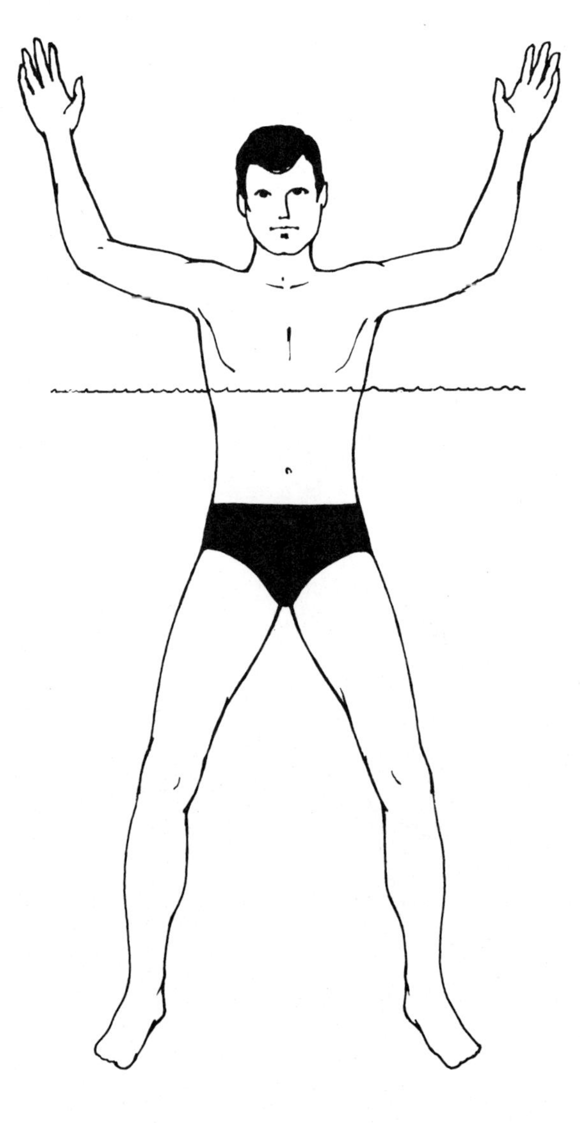

1

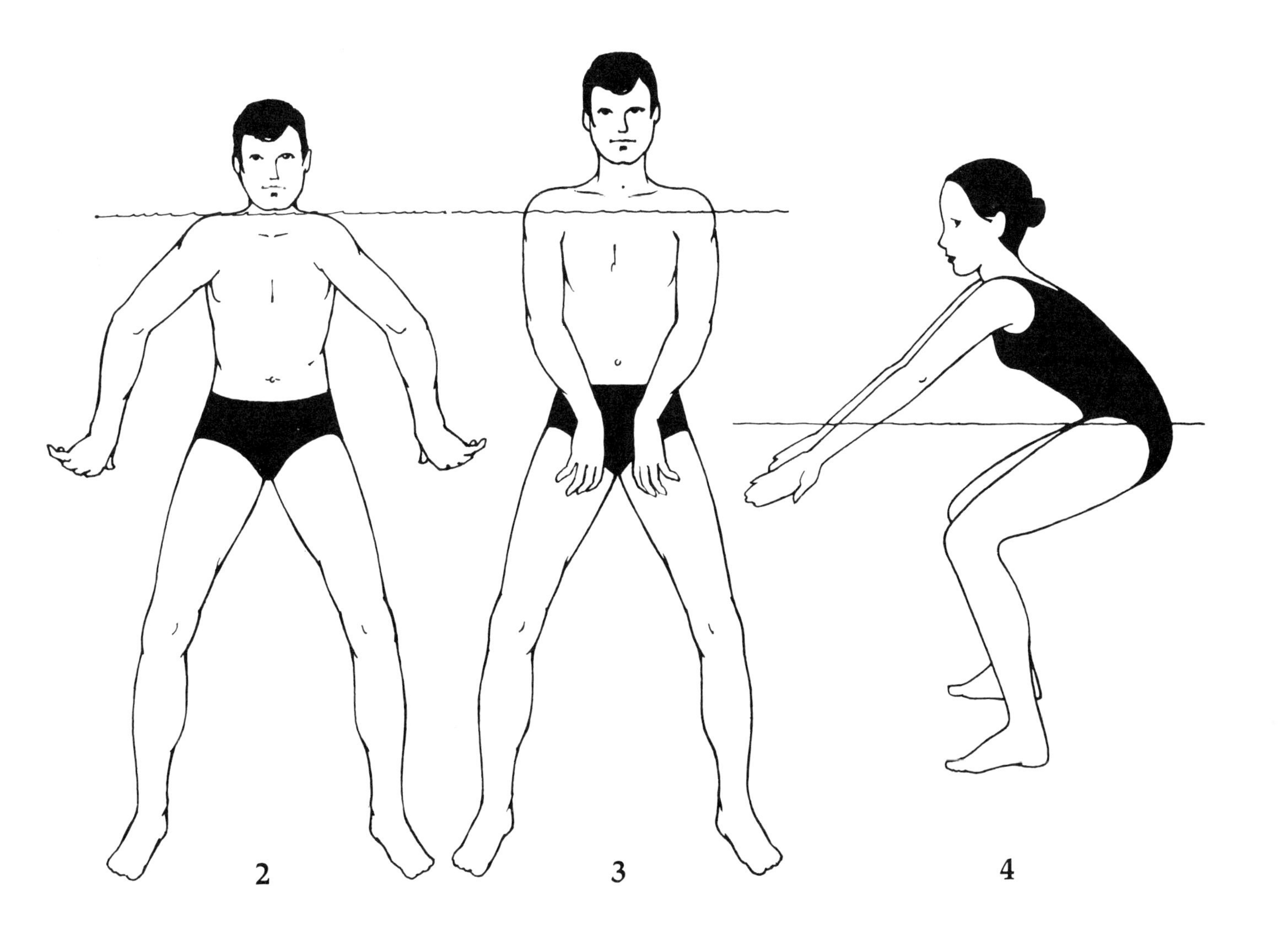
2
3
4

The Chest

The most comprehensive exercises for the bust line generally are to be found in swimming, but the strokes have different effects. Firstly, the rib-cage is uplifted by swimming, to give a firm foundation for the breasts. The crawl builds up the pectoral muscles beneath the breasts, so improving the line of the breasts from the side view. The breaststroke widens the base of each breast, and the back-stroke tends to pull the breasts up diagonally. The best thing to do is to perform all three strokes, and for that you do not necessarily have to swim, but perform the movements of the stroke with your feet on the pool rail, or have someone hold your ankles.

You can then proceed to shape your breasts by noting what shape you need to improve; if it is *frontal*, use the breast and back-stroke; for the *side view*, use the crawl.

It is best to do these exercises without any swimming-wear, or support for the breasts because the water supports them well enough.

The effect of going from hot sun into colder water—not very cold of course, that would be too much of a shock to the system, which will achieve nothing at all—is to make the nipple come out. This is a useful point to notice because, encased in a bra for too long during the day, the nipples tend to stay retracted.

The effect of massage is to encourage blood to flow more quickly through the bust tissues—an important aid in their health and shape—since the tissues must be kept well aerated by oxygen, and the cells well nourished from the nutrients in the blood.

In addition to these exercises for the breasts, look, too, at the effects of the arm exercises which involve pushing and sweeping against water resistance. You will see how your breasts and the muscles underneath them form part of your routine breast-work.

These exercises are also good for men, since the stronger the work effort is, the greater the benefit to the lungs, the chest muscles, and the rib-cage—an important consideration for men whose jobs are sedentary, since the musculature in this part of the human body is powerful and needs to be worked.

The Back

The chief drawback we have in our engineering is that the spinal column was evolved, to carry our weight when we were on all fours. As we progressed in our history from the four-legged to the upright stance there was some redistribution of weight necessary, with longer legs and a wider pelvic girdle. The stresses the spinal column receives are particularly bad in the middle and lower back, where, as we get tired, the arch becomes more and more pronounced, more concave, so that the tough cushion discs between the vertebrae can get pushed out, rather on the principle of the discs in tiddleywinks, though of course the process is much more slow.

Sitting makes the problem worse, because not only are the discs put under this strain, but the muscles lying alongside the spinal column are not exercised. A slipped disc can occur, but long before this many people complain of tired and aching backs.

The exercises here are specially designed to help counteract these developments, but of course the many movements in the book all help the strengthening of this important area.

To strengthen the back muscles in the vulnerable areas just discussed you need to practise stretching, for which water provides the ideal medium. Varying the kind of stroke you do in swimming is important too. Use the breast-stroke, the back-stroke, and the crawl, and eventually try and master the butterfly which is ideal as a general back conditioner.

JUMPING-BACK

Put your arms akimbo in water up to your waist, legs apart, now bend down as if you were doing the standing long jump. Now try to jump. The effort you make here puts useful co-ordination forces upon your back, bending it convex then concave. If you find this too difficult, try water up to your knees at first.

LEAPER

If you jump off the side of a swimming-pool into deep water, trying to hit the water with your feet flat, there will be a slight shock up your back. If you keep your hands over your head, your feet pointed, you will slide into the water in a graceful curve, showing that you are keeping your back flexibly arched.

ROCKET

Here you jump out into the water from the side, but do a half turn in the air, and then enter the water as in 'leaper'. This time you get the benefit of the twisting exercise as well as the benefits of 'leapér'. Repeat twisting in the opposite direction.

DIVER

The shock of diving into water, like a racing swimmer at the start of a race, is particularly powerful in strengthening the back muscles alongside the spinal column. At first do it from a stationary position, gently. As time goes on take a sprint to the side of the pool and dive in at great speed. Once you have mastered this technique your strength will be sufficient for you to take the daily abuses of sitting, and being cooped up in offices, in your stride.

HIGH DIVER

The effect of diving from a board into water vertically is first felt on the outstretched arms, so that there is a jack-knife effect on the back. It follows therefore that if you keep your back naturally arched, it has to work hard to keep this form as you enter the water. Work through the other exercises before you lead up to this, and then only do it from a small height. In general, anything above ten feet, which you will eventually aspire to, should be left to expert divers.

THE DOLPHIN

An excellent shapener and strengthener of the back is shown in **9**, where you start on the side of a swimming-pool, holding on to the bar. Push off, using power in your wrists, arch your back backwards, and push out your toes, as shown in **10**. Continue the motion as shown in **11** until you are flat on the surface of the water **12**. Then come back to the original position by reverse movements, through **11**, **10** to **9**. This is excellent for the tummy, top of the thighs, the chest and bust and the back. Five or 7 repetitions will be quite enough to make you aware that you have muscles there that needed exercise.

You can also do this exercise in the sea if you get hold of somebody's hands; or possibly two people, one holding each hand, to hold you as you push away. Remember, you aren't pushing with your feet here but uncurling, as it were, from position 9.

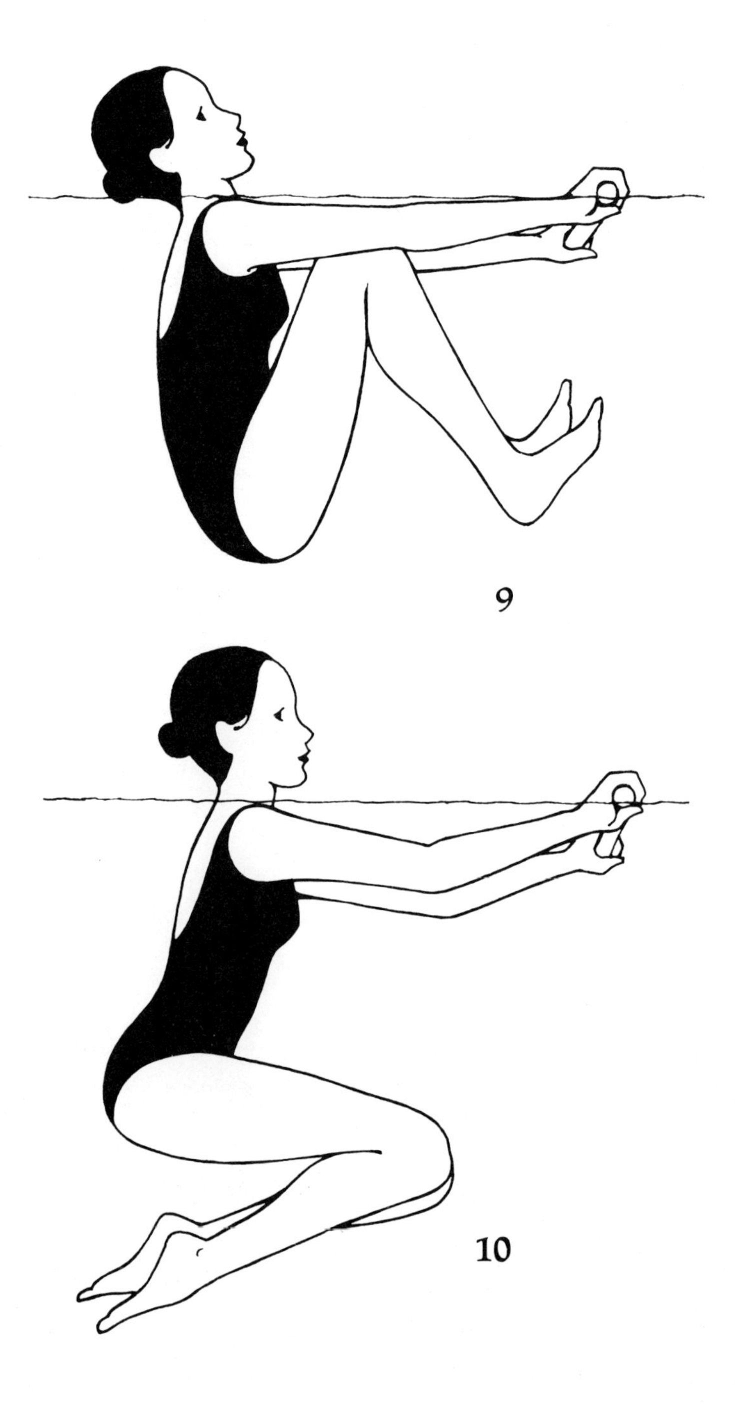

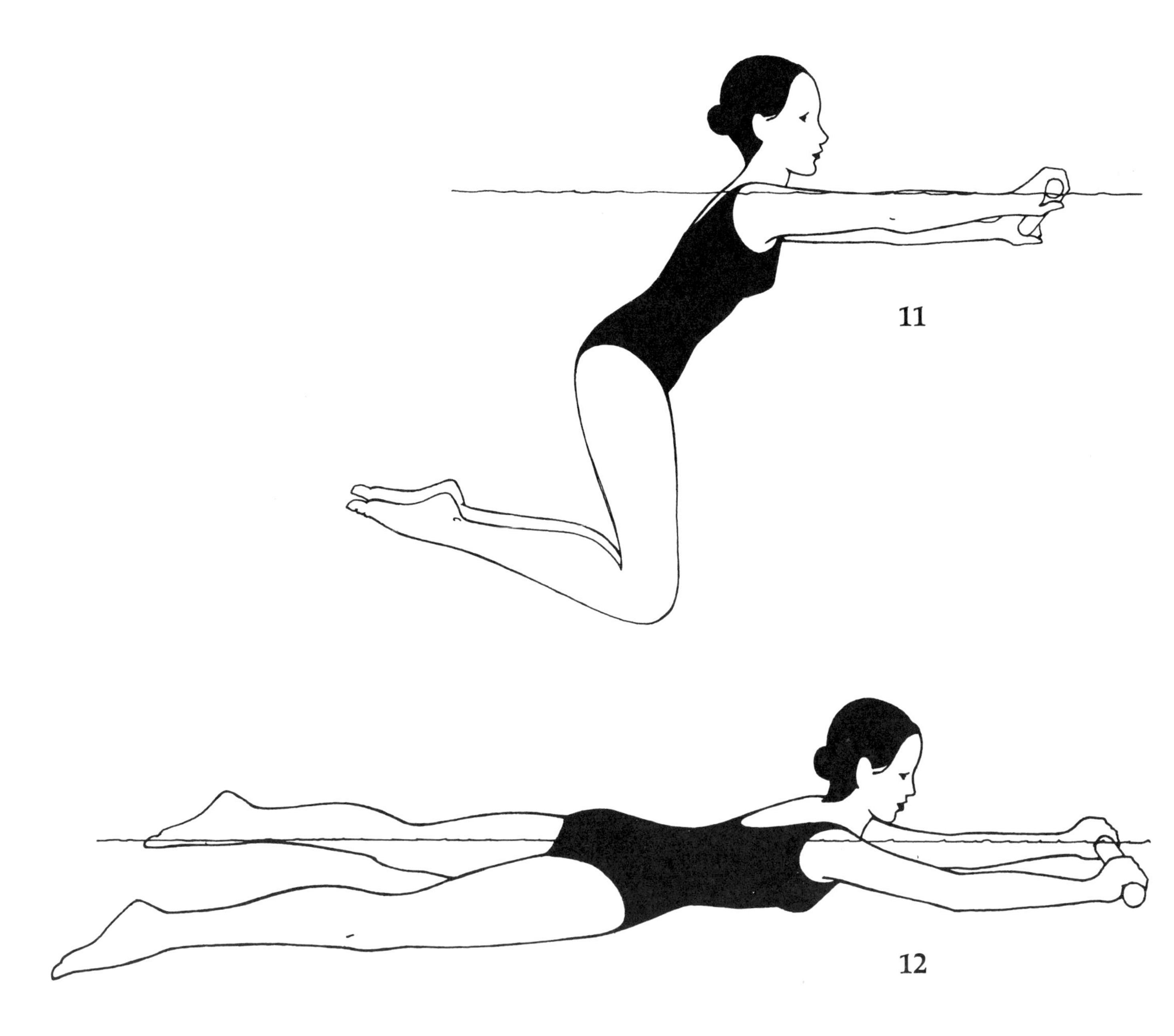
11
12

THE KELP

Another useful shaper of the upper back starts at position **13**. Your feet should be on the floor of the swimming-bath with water up to your neck. Lean out into the water with your bottom still up against the wall and push yourself back. The work done here—pulling yourself back in **14**—is against the water, as you pull against it. The harder you pull, the quicker you pull, the more pressure there is. Then push yourself out into position **13** again. It is best for this exercise to be done with the water at the level shown in **13**, but for a far more advanced exercise it can be done in much deeper water.

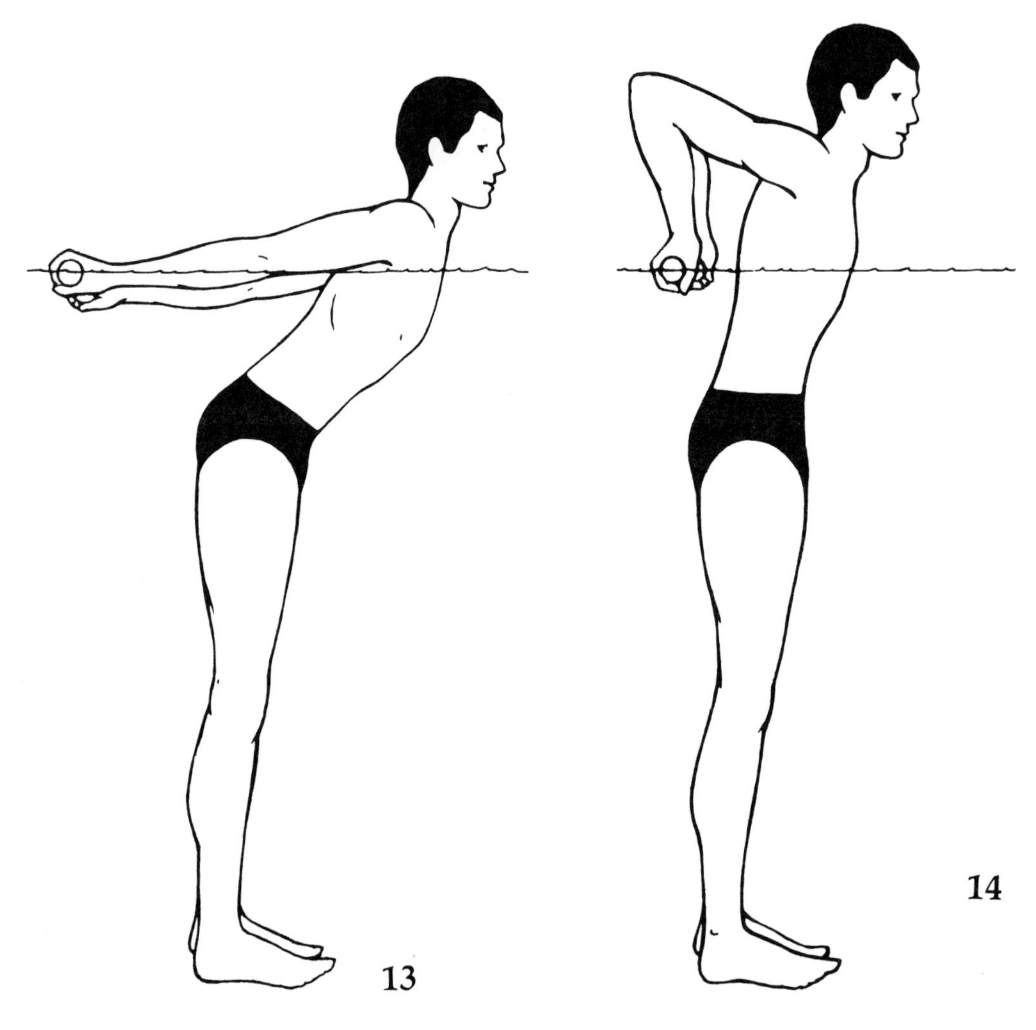

THE STARFISH

For stretching your back try floating in 'the starfish' position—with your arms and legs fully stretched and as wide apart as possible.

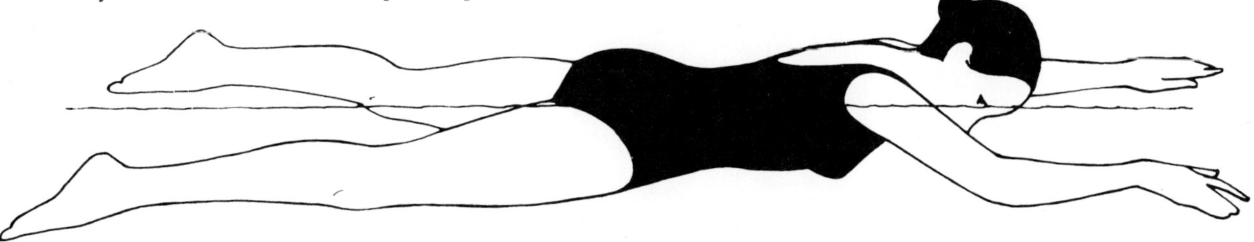

Chapter Eight

HOW TO FEEL GOOD

HOW TO FEEL GOOD

Stress is the modern curse, affecting every one of us in some way or another. Although stress claims many victims, it is not generally understood that much of our stress is stored in our bodies, making us feel bad.

When you are trying to meet a deadline you push yourself hard to reach it, but as you become tensed up you unconsciously start to contract other muscles, which have nothing to do with what you are doing. These muscles vary in different people, but the usual areas are the jaw, the throat, the shoulders, the area between the shoulder blades, and the buttocks.

These tensions can usually be lost when you relax after work, but some people carry them on to the next day, and the next, so that the tensions spread often to the tummy (which can eventually lead to ulcers), to the inside of the thighs, and the pelvic floor.

When you are stressed it often shows up in your inability to feel good sexually and otherwise. The muscles in the sensitive part of your body, where the nerves are particularly responsive to sexual needs, become bunched and tense and prevent you from enjoying sex as satisfactorily as you would wish. If you do not feel satisfied, relaxed and happy after lovemaking you are being cheated, or are cheating yourself, no matter what your age—sixteen or sixty-six. It amazes me that so many people think they can have a complex set of organs with special needs of action and stimulus and ignore them, and yet somehow lead a happy life. THEY CAN'T.

STRESS ▸ TENSION ▸ BAD SEX

BAD SEX ▸ TENSION ▸ STRESS

but consider swimming (water exercises)

RELAXATION ▸ GOOD SEX

▸ RELAXATION

The exercises that follow are specifically designed to break down the tensions discussed in this chapter.

THE PELVIS

The muscles in the pelvic floor which cup the soft organs of your abdomen should be nicely relaxed. In many women, however, they are persistently tense, either from stress or sexual hang-ups. After a tiring day they often feel hard and rindy on the outer edges, when they should be soft and springy.

Now that we know where the muscles are supposed to be relaxed, we also need to know the muscles which should be firm, but which are all too often flabby; the outer ones of the tummy, thighs and buttocks. Women with their insides knotted up and their outsides slack are not going to be healthy or have fine bodies. The same applies to men, of course, and is a prime cause of impotence and sexual inadequacy.

THE ACROBAT

A good general exercise which also exercises the hips is shown in the beginning position in **1** where you stand in a swimming-bath and raise your feet up into position **2** holding hard on to the bar and then through **3** to **4**. Push yourself up as hard as you can, first allowing the back to swing backwards as shown in **4** then making the legs straighten out as in **5** so that in **6** you are coming away from the wall of the bath. Repeat this with the legs further and further apart in position **2.**

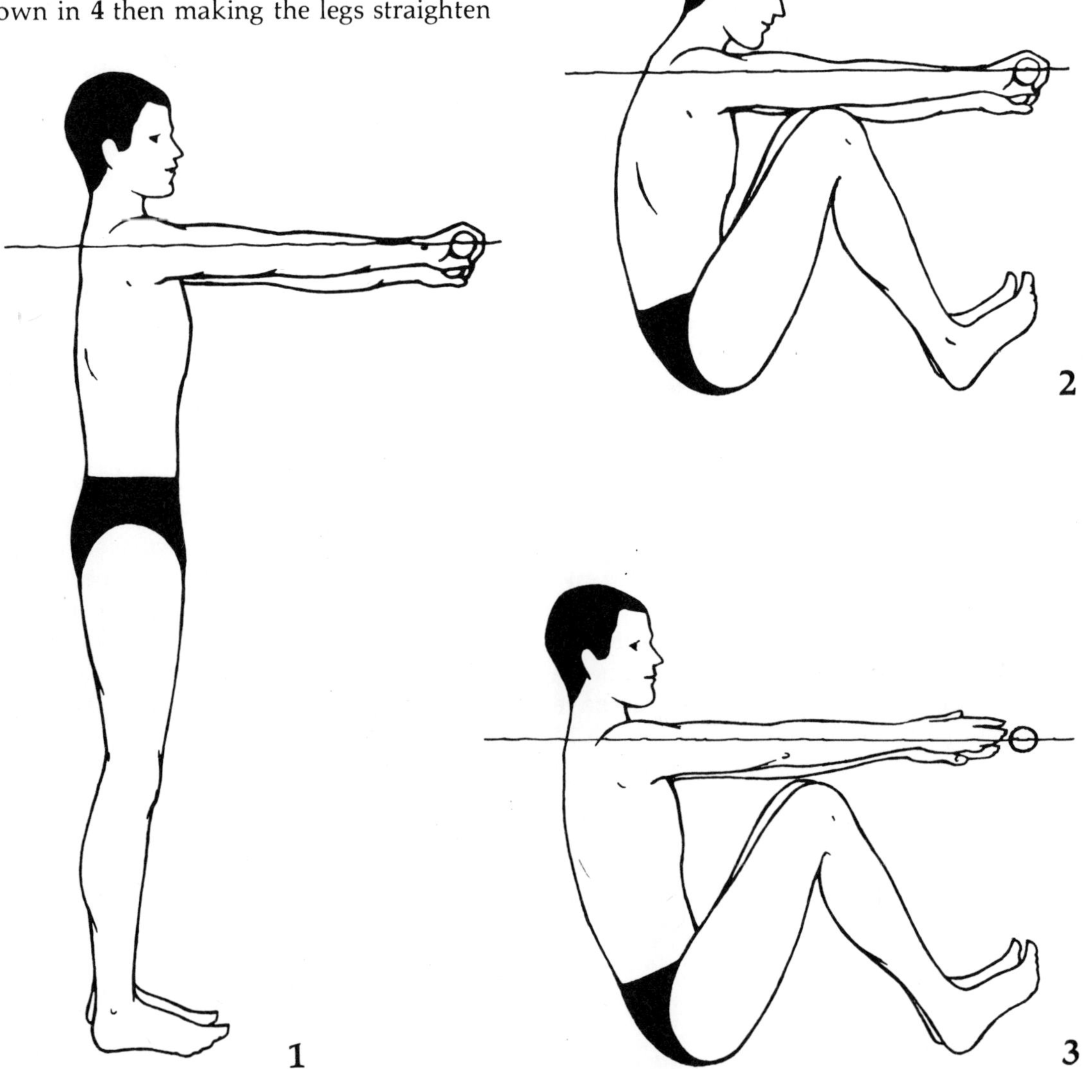

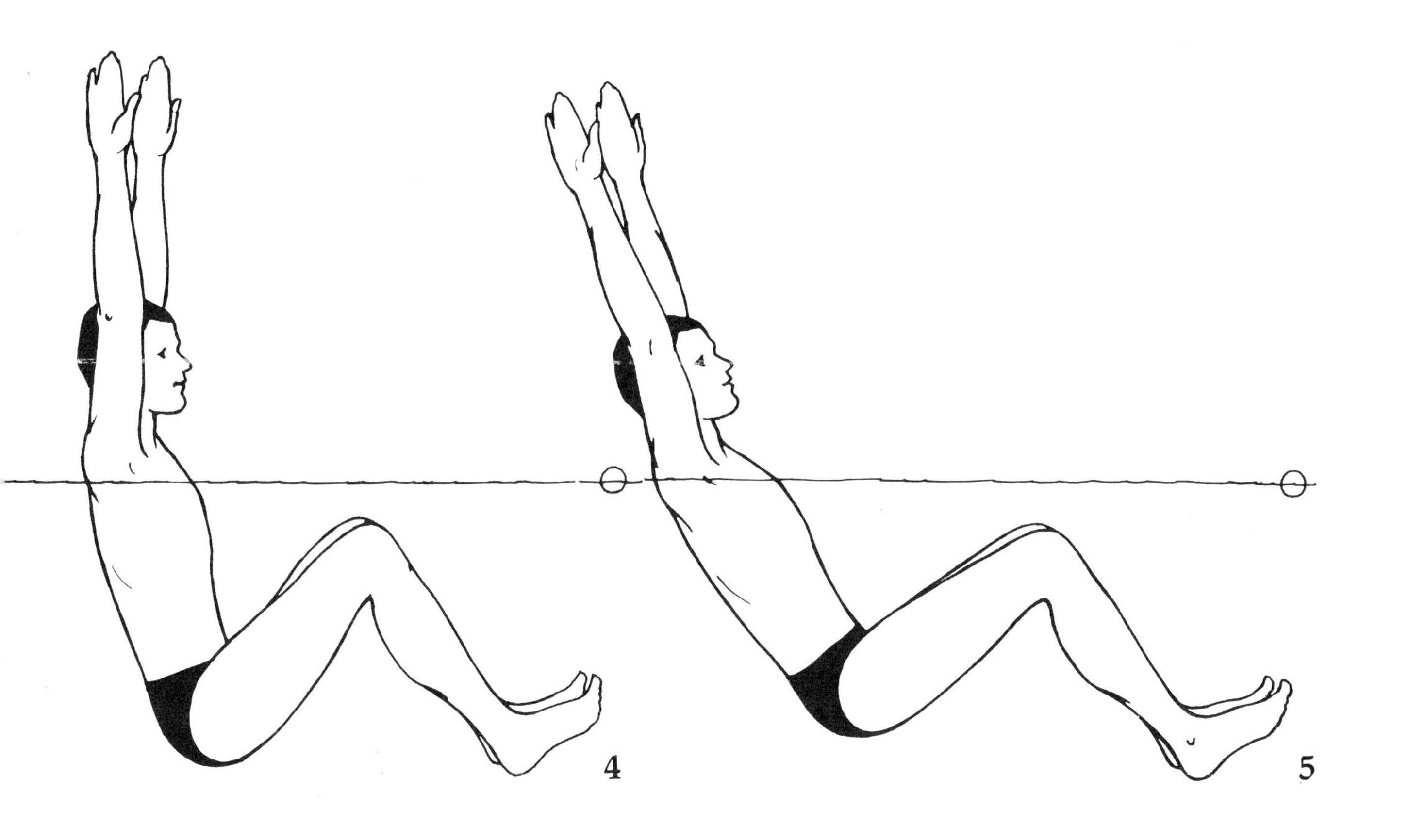
4
5

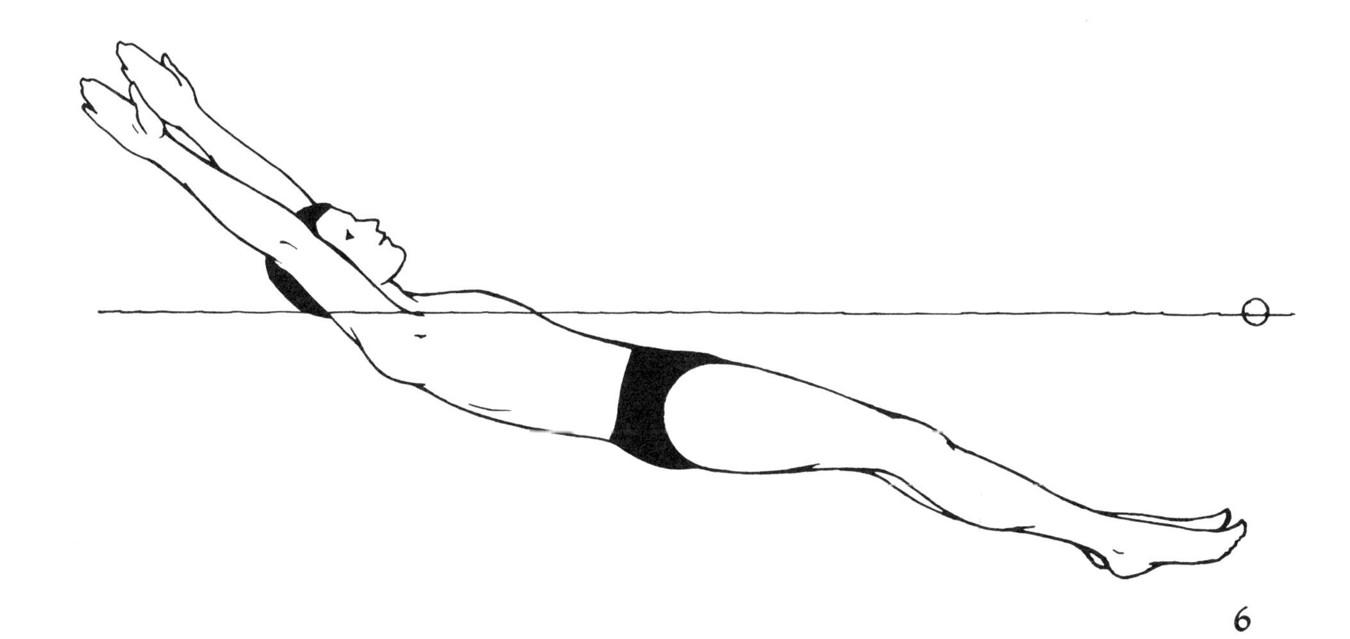
6

THE CAT

You may have seen cats use a stretching exercise like the one shown in **7** and they don't have to worry much about their feline grace. Take up the position shown, in about a foot of water, and then raise one leg off the floor, keeping it straight, and hold for a count of seven, then relax. Repeat with the other leg. Continue in this way, all the time working the legs further and further apart. You may find this difficult to do at first, but when you become proficient you can try this in the shallow end of the pool, holding on to the bar.

A variation on this is to take up position **8**, again in about a foot of water, and move your leg forward and backward over the leg that is lying flat, as shown in **9**. Then, as you get used to that, move it from **9** to position **10**. As time goes on, you'll get better and better at it and you'll feel the joints of the hip and any tightness in the tummy give way. It's important of course to do this in reasonably warm water. If you are lucky enough you may have a large bath tub in which you can do this exercise sitting in warm water up to about the hip. It is extremely good for you as warm water helps the blood flow in the skin and through the inner organs, particularly those in the lower abdomen. Consequently this is a very relaxing exercise in itself.

As far as the beauty effects of these exercises are concerned, the stretching exercises that we've described from **7** to **10** are excellent for the crotch and the lower part of the tummy, and also for the junction of the thigh with the hip—areas which are usually extremely difficult to exercise. I repeat that it is best to do the exercises in warm, not cold, water. The advantage in doing them in water is that the partial weightlessness you can achieve enables you to concentrate more on the joints. When you get better at the exercise you can move into deeper water, say up to the navel.

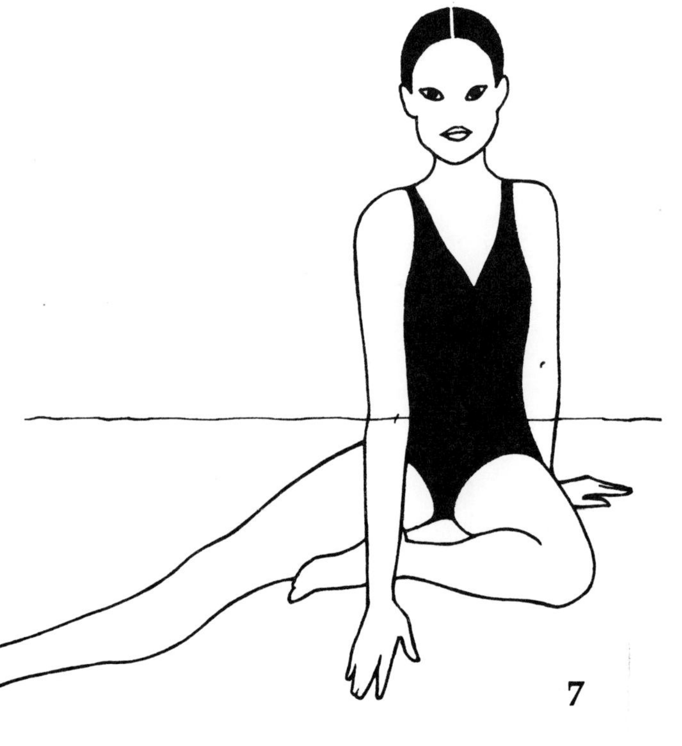

7

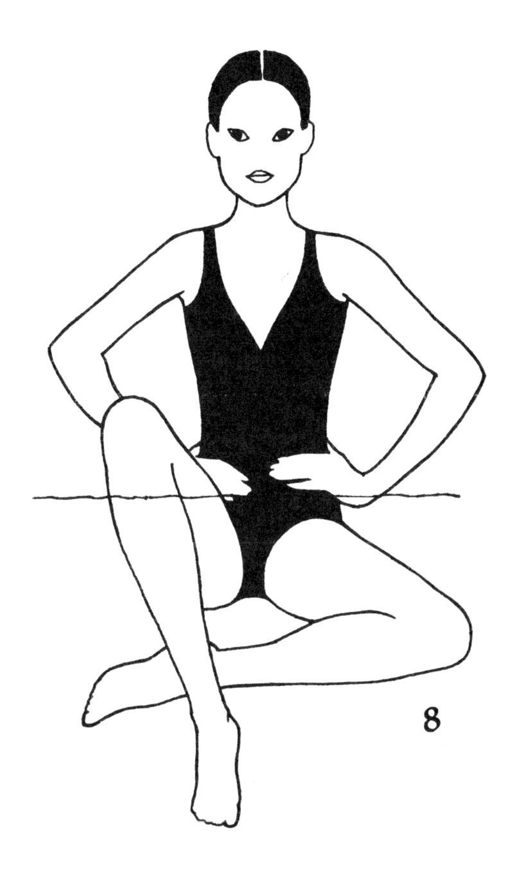

8

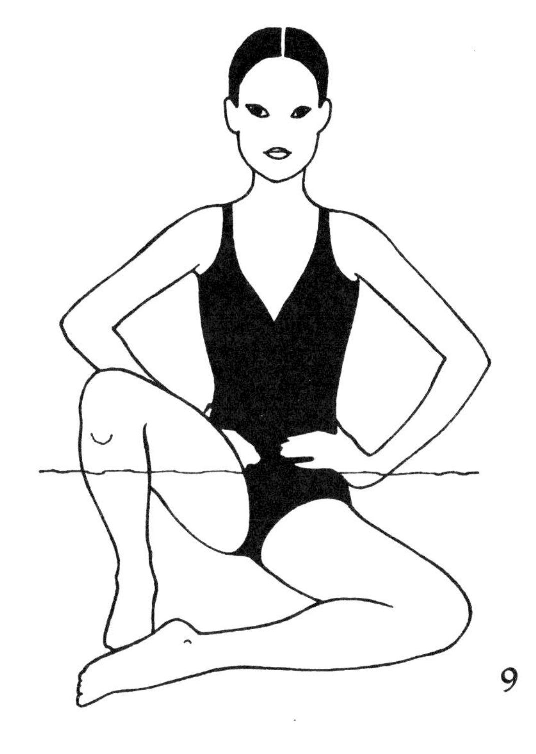

9

THE SEA URCHIN

The position in **11** should be carried out in water just above the knees. The idea is to stretch as much as possible, going down as deep as possible, with the hands and feet absolutely flat. You can try this exercise in the bath and shower too.

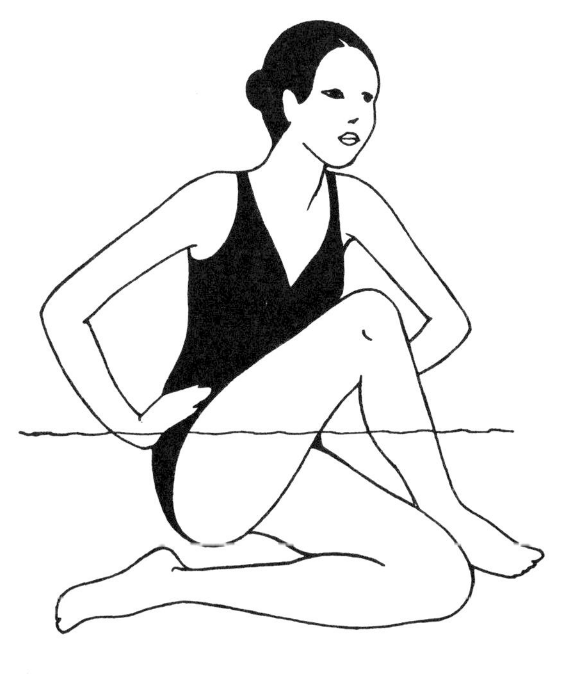

10

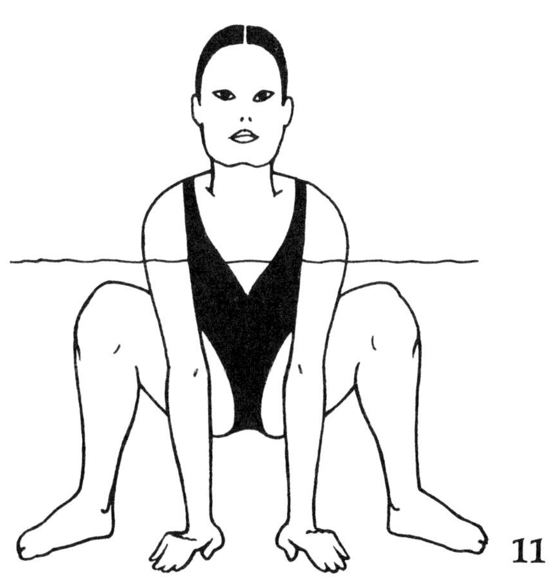

11

THE TWO-STEP

At first you will find that you will be unable to take up the position shown in **11**, in which case try moving on to the next position, **12**, which you start with water to the depth of about a foot, and your feet together. Move one leg over the other as shown in **13** and then in front of the other, **14**. Now alternate the other leg. This is a very good exercise because as you increase the level of the water your weight is increasingly taken up and you have to stretch more and more to keep the top part of the body out of the water. Also, the push against the water enables the outside of the thighs to be exercised. This is a useful exercise for the bath.

From **14** you can move on to position **15** with the legs as wide apart as possible, and the hands interlaced as shown. Press very hard on your hands, one against the other, exhale and pull your tummy in as far as possible. You should do this in water a little above your waist so that when you relax and breathe in and relax your arms, you get a push against the water. Once you become proficient at this you will find you can get ripples moving around you very easily. At first, attempt it gently to avoid pulling muscles which have been inactive for a long time.

The foregoing exercises, from **1** to **15,** can all be as effectively done by men as by women. In general, they are useful for increasing the flow of blood into those areas which are usually associated with sexual excitement. For women in particular they are extremely good figure formers, while men

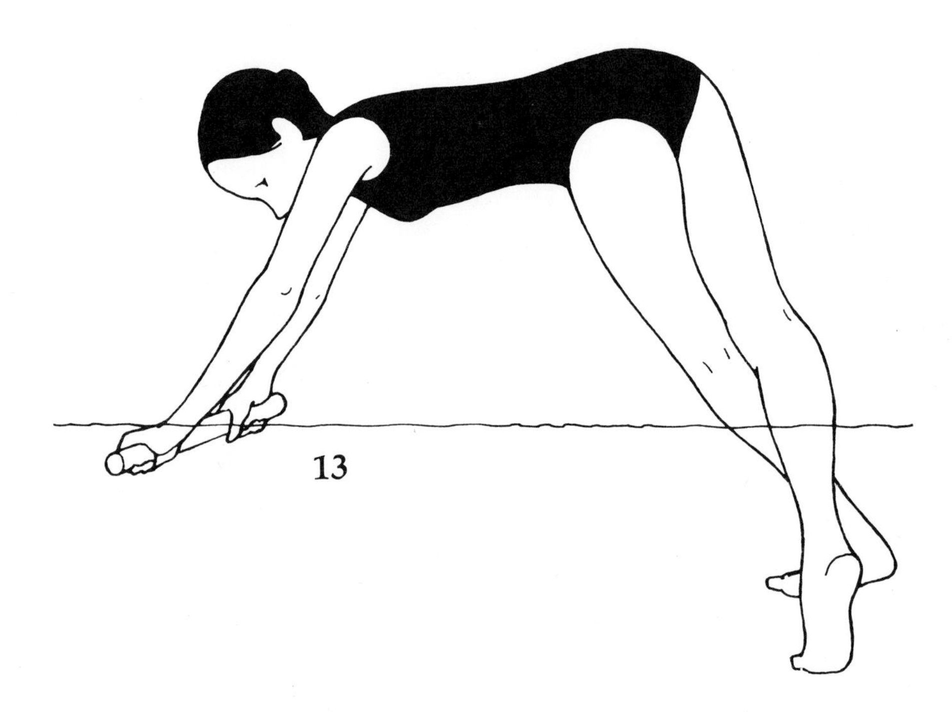
13

can use them for stretching ligaments which might otherwise get rather unexercised as the years go by. So, when I call these sexual exercises I mean this in the fullest sense. They improve the flow of blood in the areas which should have a high blood level, and they utilise areas of the body which should be very fit for happy sexual relationships. Moreover, they turn you on to your body, should you need it, because in these exercises you should feel definite changes in your sensations, getting a warm pleasurable feeling as the exercise increases. As I emphasised, warm water can help in this.

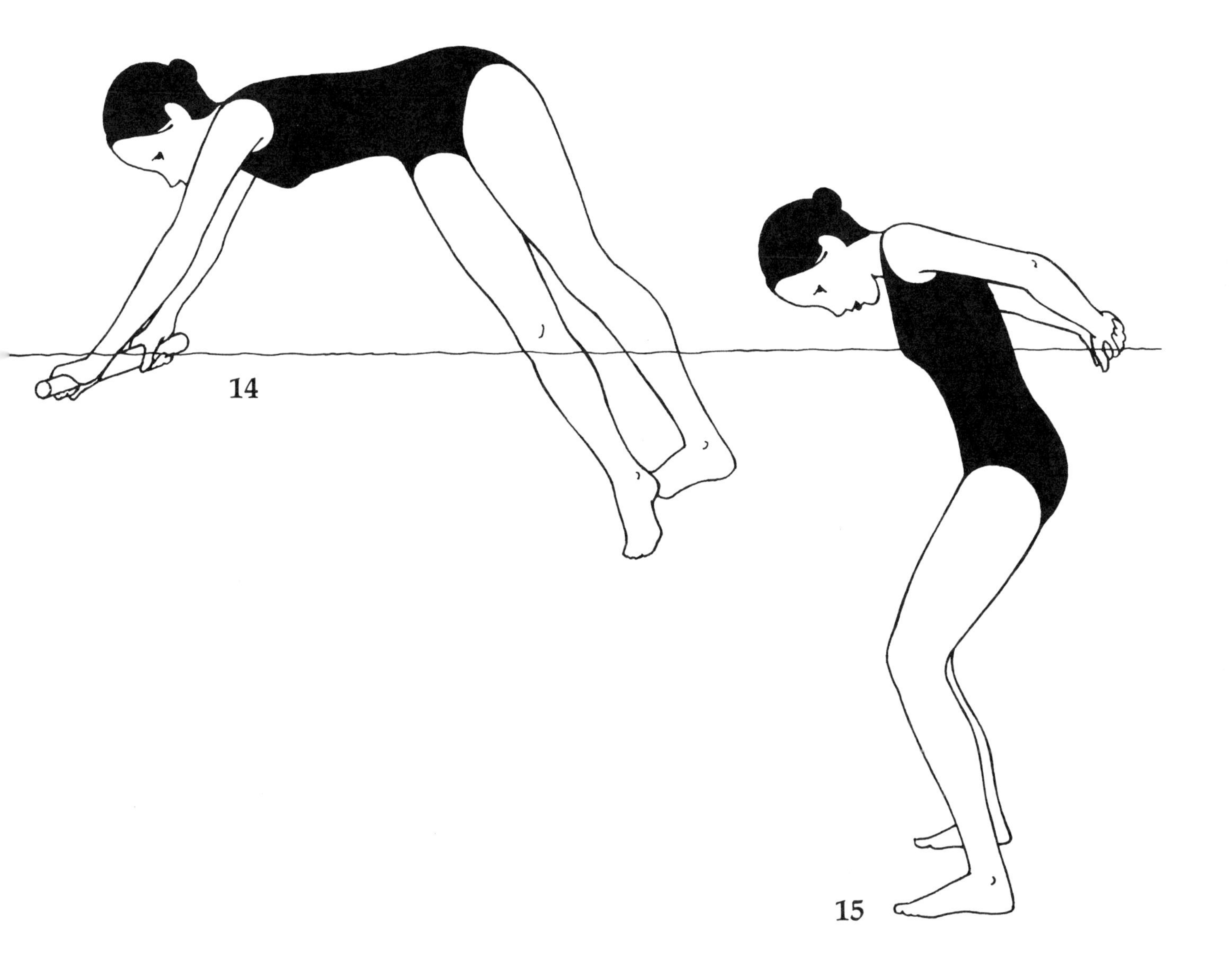

There now follows a series of advanced exercises which are best practised first on dry land. In the water you should not attempt them unless you are an extremely good swimmer.

These exercises were specifically designed for women but they can be done by men. When doing them in water, always have somebody supporting you, or near you in the water: not merely on the side of the swimming-pool but *actually with you in the water.* Many of them can be done in the bath at home, or just after a warm shower. If you are lucky enough to have a large bath in which you can lie out in warm water in the way described, they can be done very easily with a friend. They are well worth attempting to do.

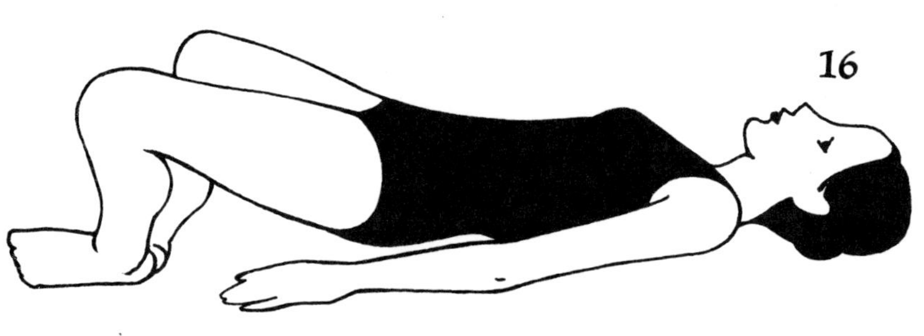

16

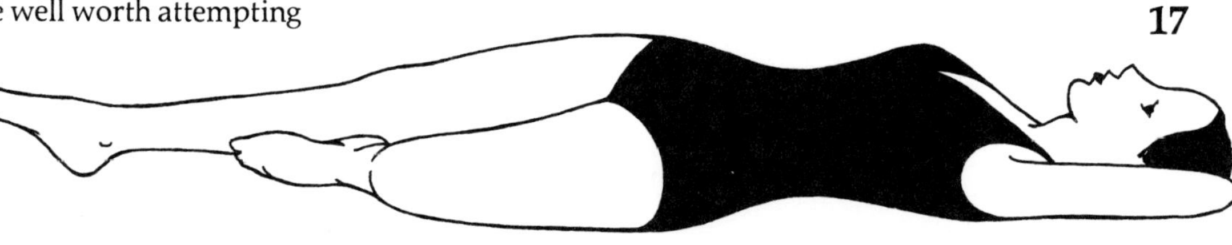

17

THE MARINA

Take up position **16**. If you are doing this in water (warm, of course), it shouldn't be deeper than about six inches. Press the feet together and let the legs fall open under their own weight. Stay in that position, breathing gently. This is a very good position for the massage of the tummy.

Now let your legs slide out and let one leg be opposed to the other as shown in drawing **17**, then press one leg into the other. Press gently at first, otherwise you'll experience slight twinges from a large tendon on the inside of the leg. Press for a few moments, relax, breathe, press again. From there you can reach position **18** where again you use a technique of pressing the feet together in the position shown. This, too, is an excellent position for massage on the inside of the thighs and along the tummy up to the neck.

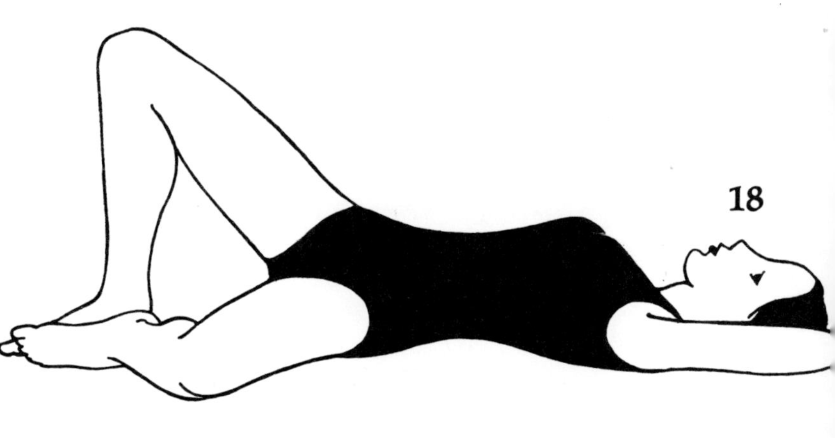

18

THE SEA-HORSE

Turn over into position **19**. *This exercise must be done in water deep enough to support your whole weight* and only when you have done all these exercises on dry land first of all, *and* are an excellent swimmer, *and* have somebody with you.

But on the dry land, say just after a shower, position **19** is excellent. Press down on the hands by the legs in the position shown, then change over legs. The idea is to stretch and hold your breath, hold the position with a considerable amount of tension then let your breath out and relax. Do this several times.

THE LILY

Move on to position **20** which is marvellous when done in the bath, and follow the same technique of breathing in and holding the breath as you press your feet together and raise your pubic arch as high as possible. Press as hard as you can, breathe in, hold until you are tired, then relax. Repeat until you feel a definite sensation of relaxation.

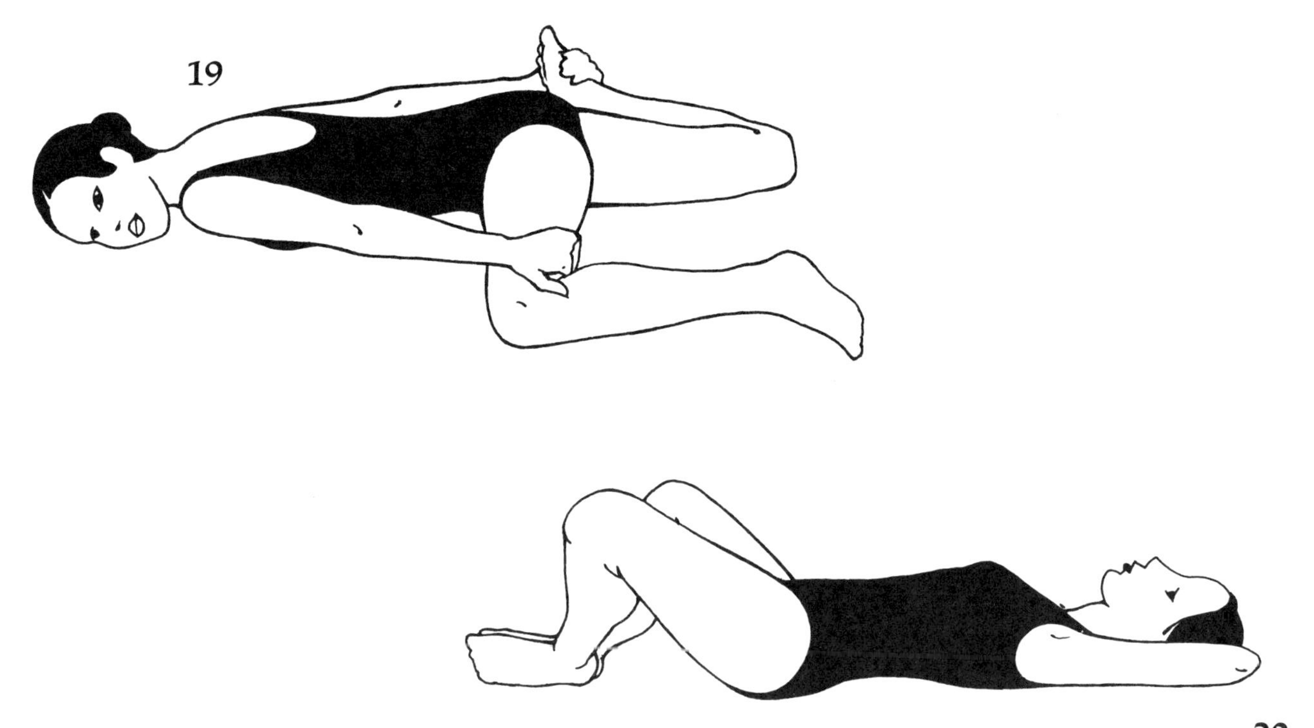

20

THE SWAY

Move on to position **21**. This is a good exercise for the hips, as most of these exercises are. Twist the body as far to the left as you can, as shown in position **22**, then as far to the right. This is one exercise that you can do in, say, 18 inches of water, just covering your hips so that the effect on the waist is much more exaggerated because of the pressure against the water.

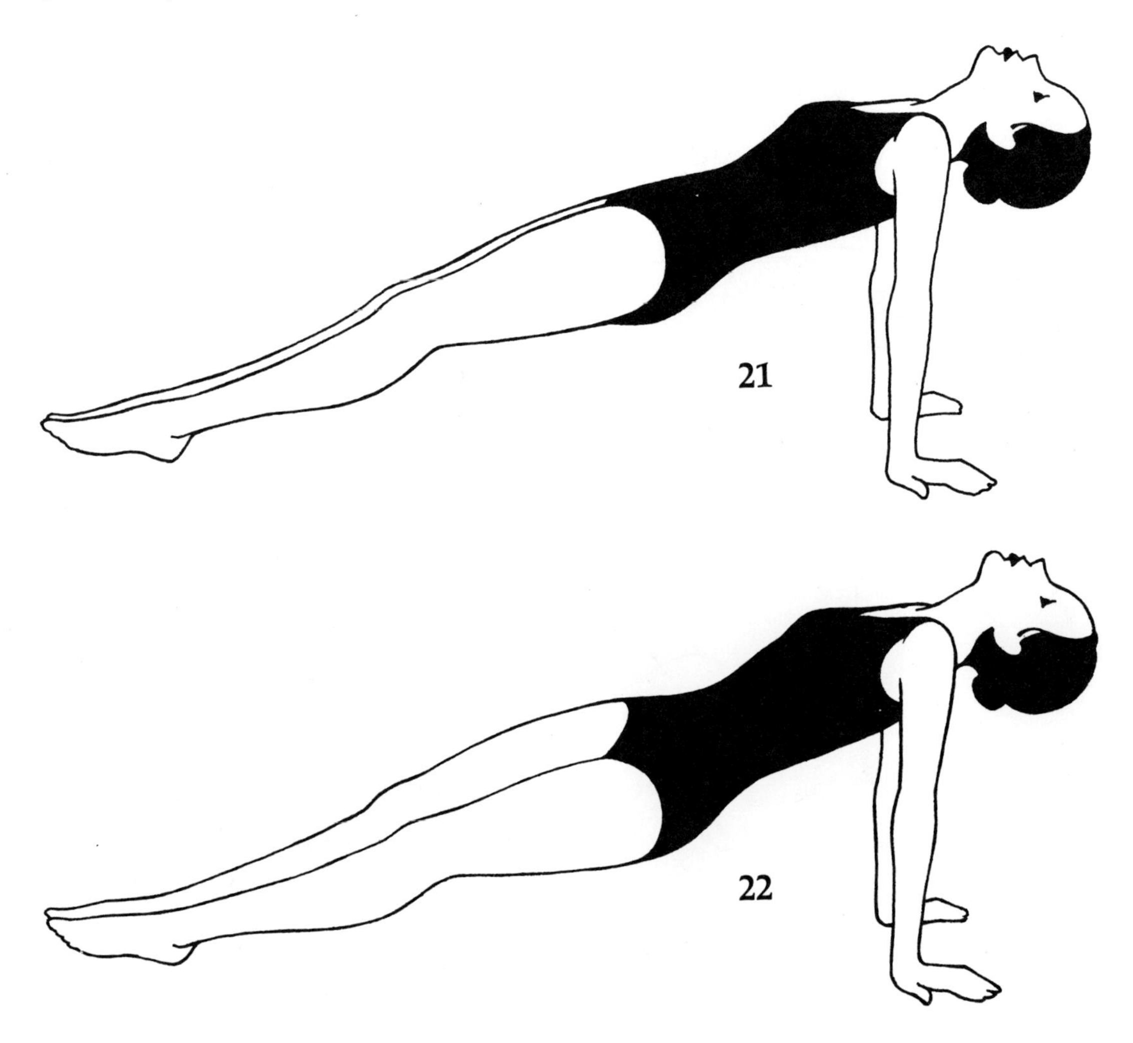

THE CLAMP

You then move to position **23** pressing against the legs and buttocks with the hands and gradually changing this so that the legs are further and further apart. A variation of this is to move into **24** where you actually pull your legs towards you as near to your tummy as you can.

THE WHIRLPOOL

Move into position **25** and perform circles with each leg at the same time, first anti-clockwise, then clockwise.

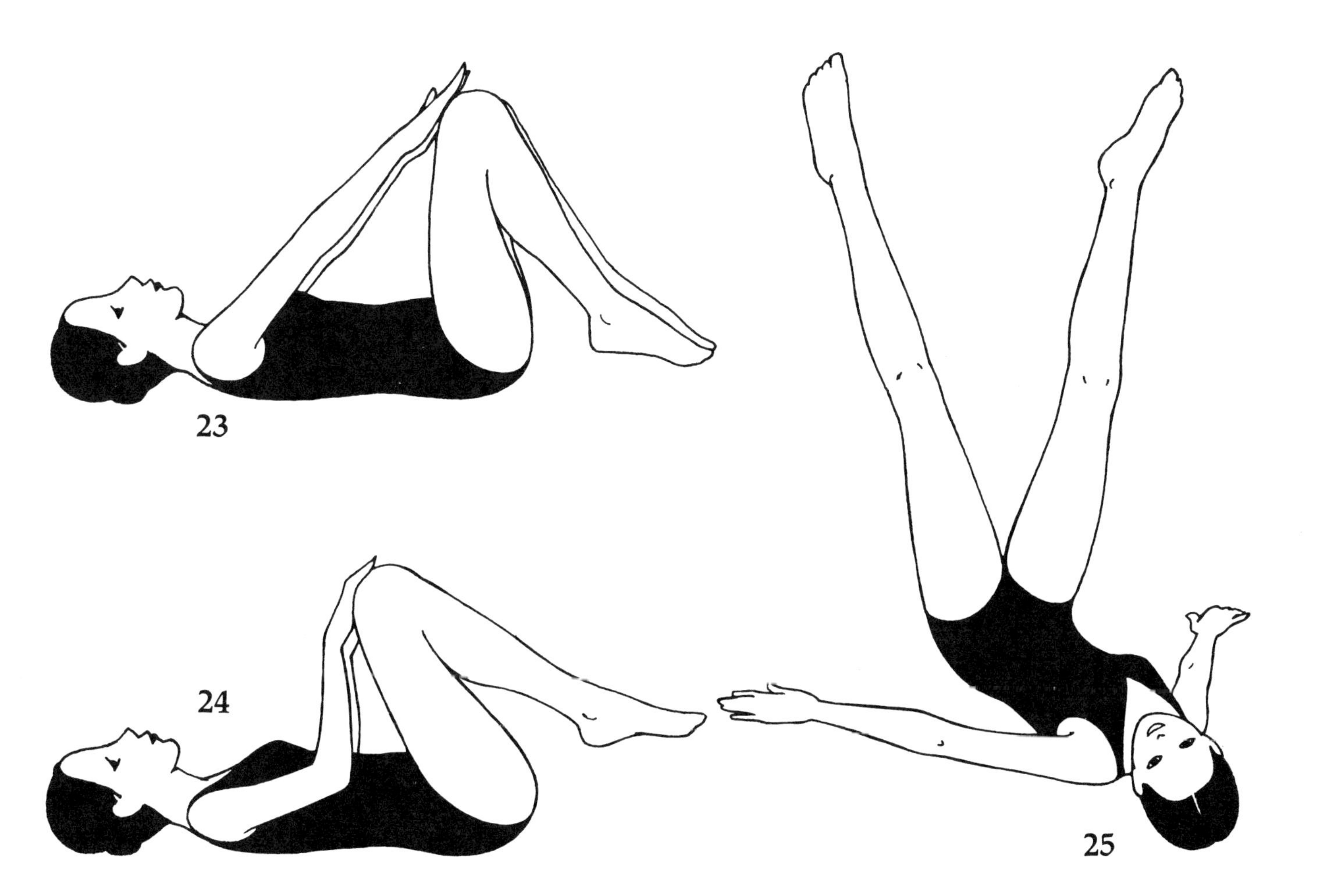

THE CRAB

Then you can move on to position **26**. The technique here is to press the feet together, legs as far apart as possible, pull hard on the ankles, breathe in, stretch out as far as you can, hold the breath, then relax. Continue until you distinctly feel relaxation between your legs.

THE CANTILEVER

Move on to **27**. Here the method is to bring the leg up towards the chest as far as you can then press the other one out as far as you can, taking your weight on your hands. Repeat for the other leg.

26

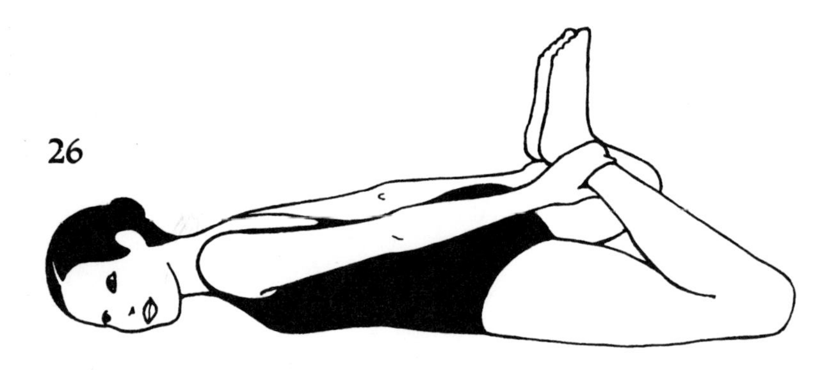

27

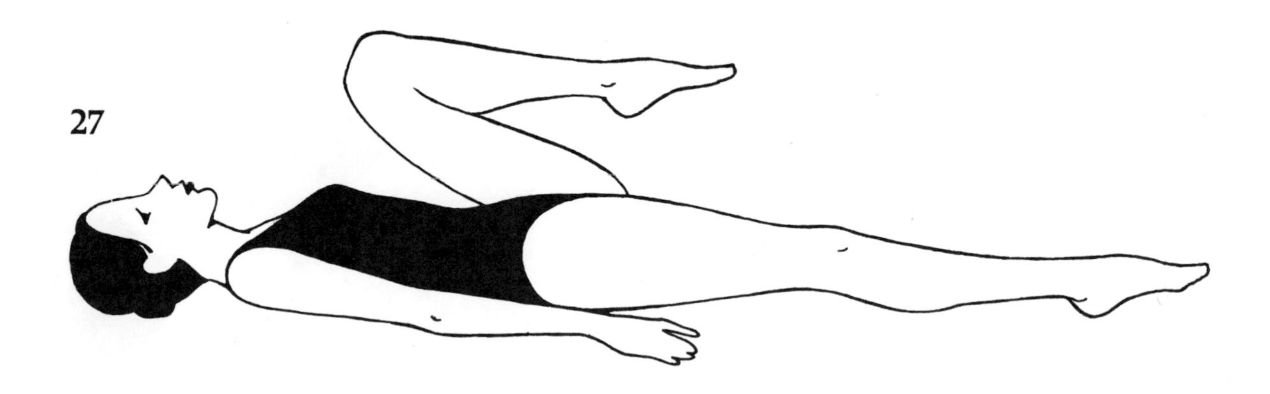

THE FROND

You then move into position **28**. Again you use the pressing technique where you press your feet together and bend your back up and press your neck against your hands. Breathe in, hold as long as you can, relax into position **29** then take the position up again until you feel a pleasant sensation.

The sequence **16** to **29** is best learned by doing each separate exercise until you have mastered it before passing on to the next. After a while you'll be able to put the exercises together into a continuous sequence, on dry land. As I have said, some of the exercises can be done in a few inches of warm water but you should only try **19, 26** or **28**, or for that matter **29**, on dry land. All these exercises can be done in water deep enough for you to swim in provided you inhale first and then try to carry out the motion. With the water supporting the weight of your body, you can concentrate on the pressings that I mentioned before.

These exercises really are very advanced and perhaps you might be happier doing them without wearing any clothes after a shower, or before a shower, or before you go to bed.

For adept exercisers the sequence **16-29** in water deep enough for total support is a kind of relaxing, sexually beneficial dance movement.

I must add that they make excellent positions for massage techniques, which are discussed in the following chapters.

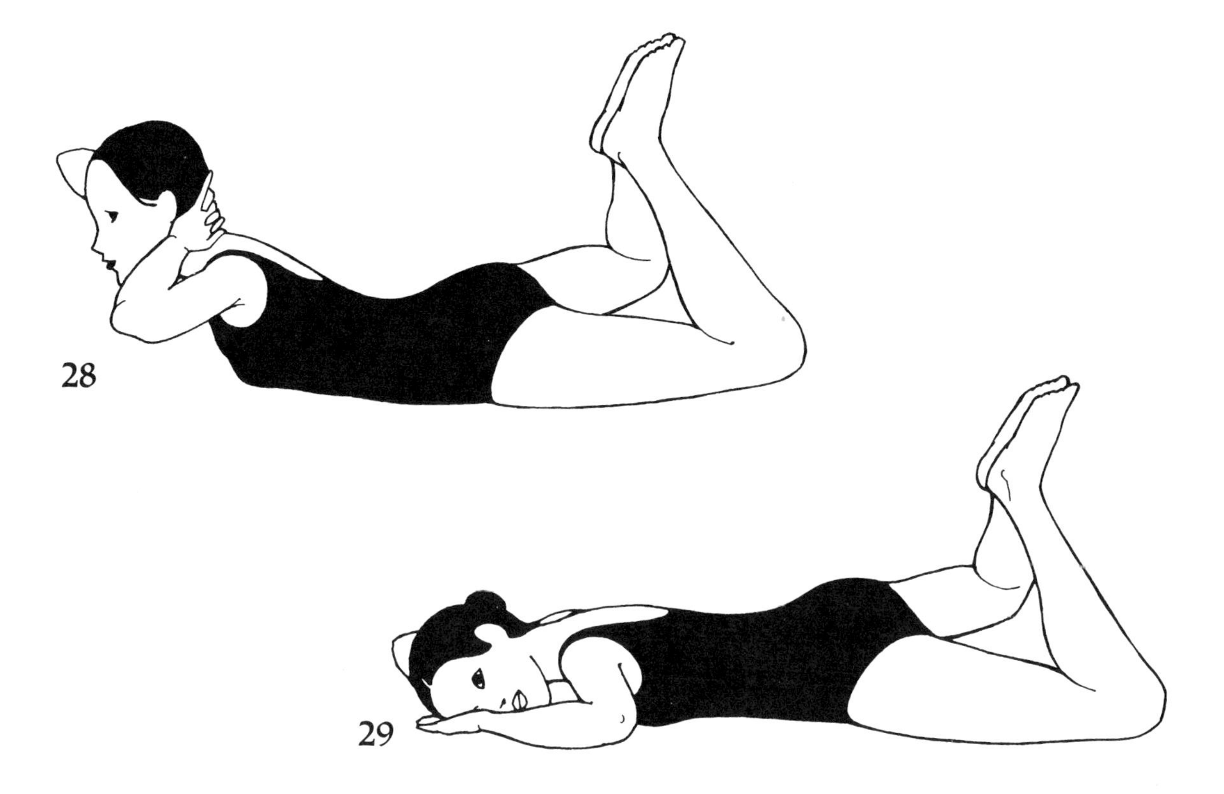

Chapter Nine

WATER MASSAGE

WATER MASSAGE

In this chapter you will find techniques for massaging yourself and also massaging your friends, and having your friends massage you. Some can be done under the shower, some can be done on the beach using the anti-sun lotions as a lubricant, while some are for work in the swimming-bath and the sea.

Massage comes in many types. The usual type practised in Europe involves stroking the skin and then working rather more deeply on the muscles; kneading them, pummelling them and pressing them.

We know that fish have along the sides of their bodies a line of sense organs, called the lateral line. Although we do not have a single line like this, there are some similarities in that we have many connections of sensitive points around the body grouped together in meridia. At this stage, it is not necessary to know individually the several hundred points that are involved as we are going to exploit those points by massaging, pressing with the finger tips, the palms of the hands and the heel of the hand areas containing these points.

Water provides an excellent medium for this because warm water especially makes the blood flow, and by lubrication helps the hands to slide easily over the skin. In all the work that follows, when a largish area is indicated use the heel of the hand to press against it; when a smaller area is involved, use the finger tips. Make sure that your finger-nails are not long enough to tear the skin.

In general, you keep up the massage until you feel the desired effect, which will be relaxing, soothing and pleasurable.

Certain areas of the body, although they are not located near the sexual organs, enable one to get sexually relaxed. This can be used as a preliminary to lovemaking rather than more athletic and, to some people, spine-chilling techniques which are all huff and puff. These methods are very gentle. They are a marvellous way of getting to know yourself, and other people. They are also excellent for health and toning effects.

Work done in several hospitals around the world has proved that stimulation of these points can cut off pain. These points have been useful for certain treatments, such as the reduction of the pain of headaches, rheumatic sprains and fatigue. Also it seems that as stimulation of the points increases the general level of vital activity of the body they are useful in shaping the figure and for losing weight.

The health and appearance of the skin is improved when blood circulation is increased in the blood vessels beneath the skin. This flow can be improved by massage, but you do not need to go to a masseur or a massage parlour. The actual motions shown can easily be carried out by you alone, or you can ask a partner to do them for you. They can be done on the beach or in the shower or in your bath. The methods that follow can improve the shape of your body and also improve muscle tone. Try them and see.

In the shower, do not use very hot water: on the other hand, never massage in very cold water.

The techniques can also be used, suitably modified by your experience, floating in the sea or in the swimming-bath. You can float on either your back or your tummy in a star shape and your partner can work over various parts of your body.

In general you should continue to do the massaging until you feel a definite increase in warmth inside your tissues, which is a pleasurable sensation.

Massage in the Shower

These are very good routines for the whole body. Follow the drawings carefully. Use warm to hot water, which helps to increase the blood flow. Use as strong a pressure with your hand as you can, but not enough to be painful.

THE ARMS

ARM AND SKIN TONER

In **1** you can see how you would space the flow of water from the shower as it cascades down your arms and down the front of your body. Start at your wrist with the palm of your hand and move firmly along the forearm, over the elbow as shown in **2** down into the armpits. Repeat several times.

Now do it to the other arm. This is also very good for getting rid of the dead skin on the elbow.

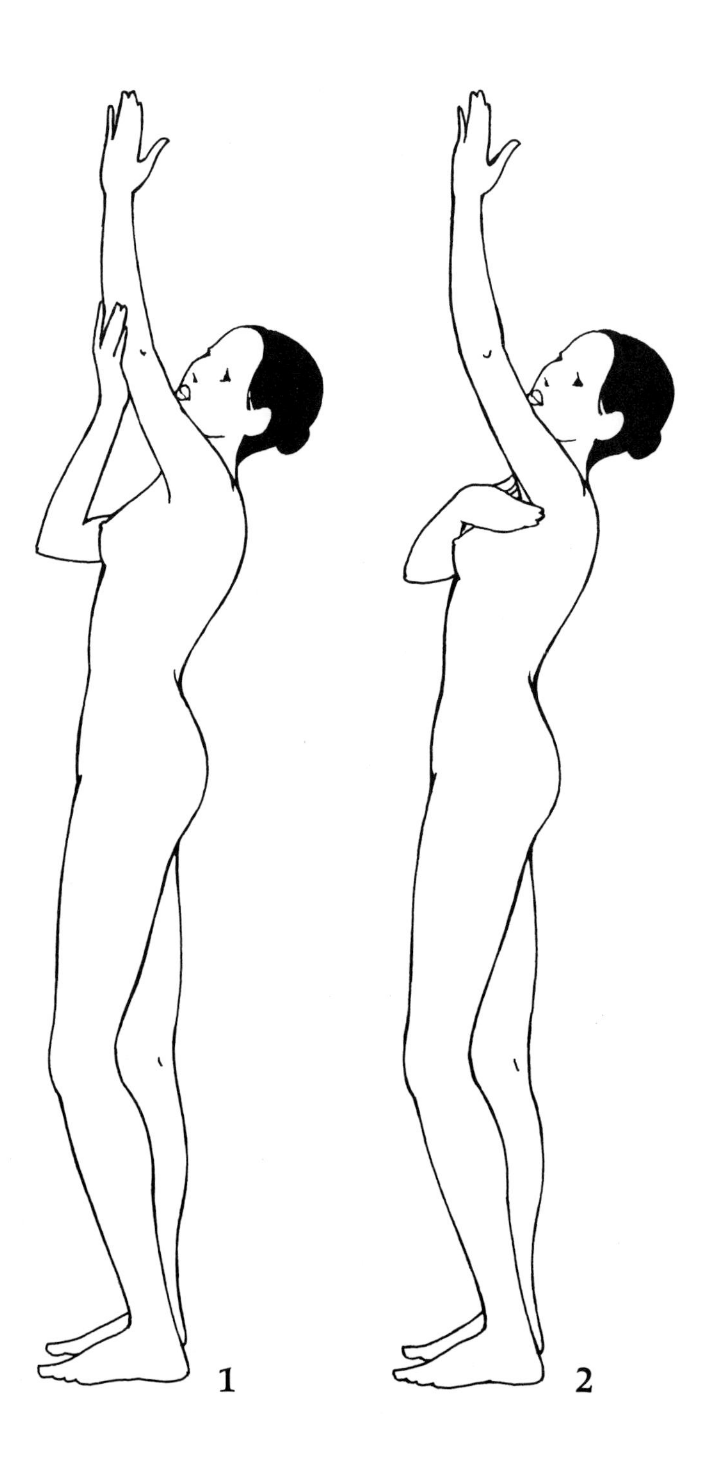

THE STOMACH

TUMMY PRESS AND PAT

For getting a good firm tone on the tummy and just above the pubic arch, use the flat palms of both hands starting as in **3**, working up towards and over the belly button, **4**. Then, with a patting motion, swop hands over and continue. Do this for at least a minute, with the water cascading on the tummy.

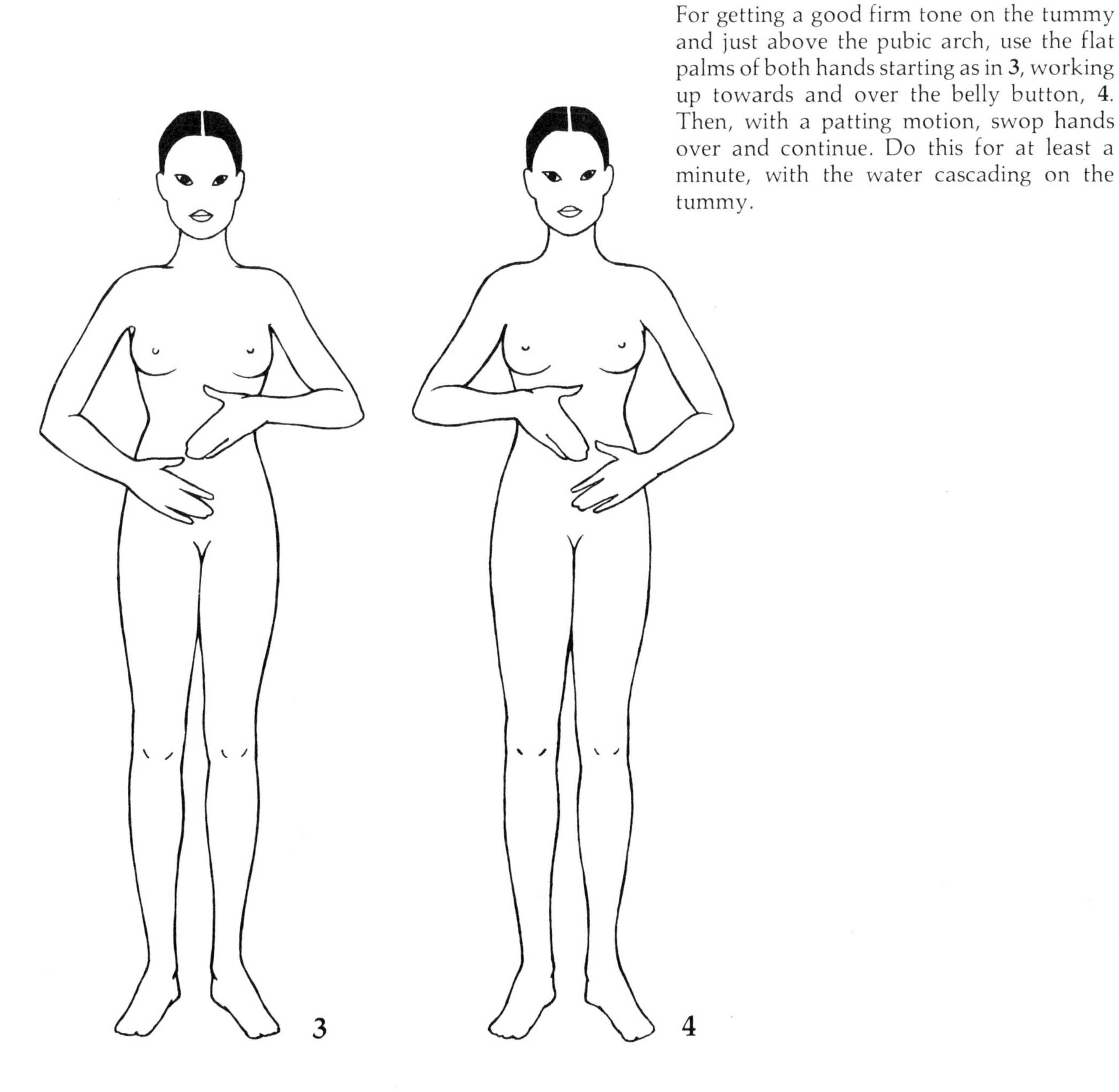

THIGHS AND WAIST

SMOOTH-LEVER

To obtain a good line for the thigh on to the waist, take up the position as shown in **5** and use the stroking-patting technique you've already learned on the tummy. Proceed, with the water as hot as you can bear it, working from the top of the thighs and draw your hands up, as shown in **6**. Press quite hard then work on the other side.

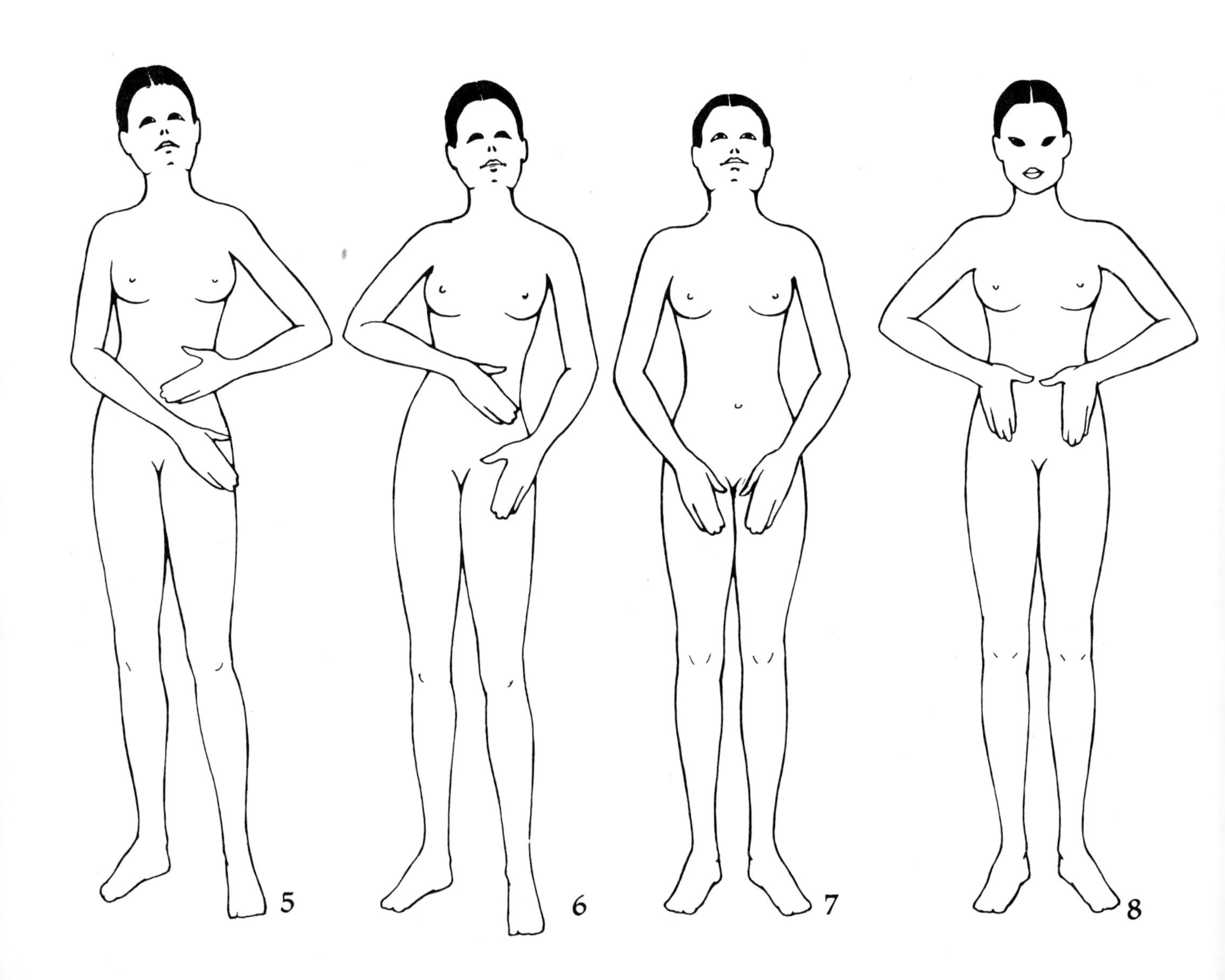

THE WHEEL

With your palms on your thighs, **7**, bring them over your tummy, **8**, up and round, **9**, right down to the top of the hips, **10**, and then sweep round on to the buttocks as shown in **11**, pressing very hard. Bring up your hands as shown in **12** over the buttocks to end at the waist. Then start the whole procedure all over again. You should do this at least five times. It produces very good smooth skin lines and guards against cellulite.

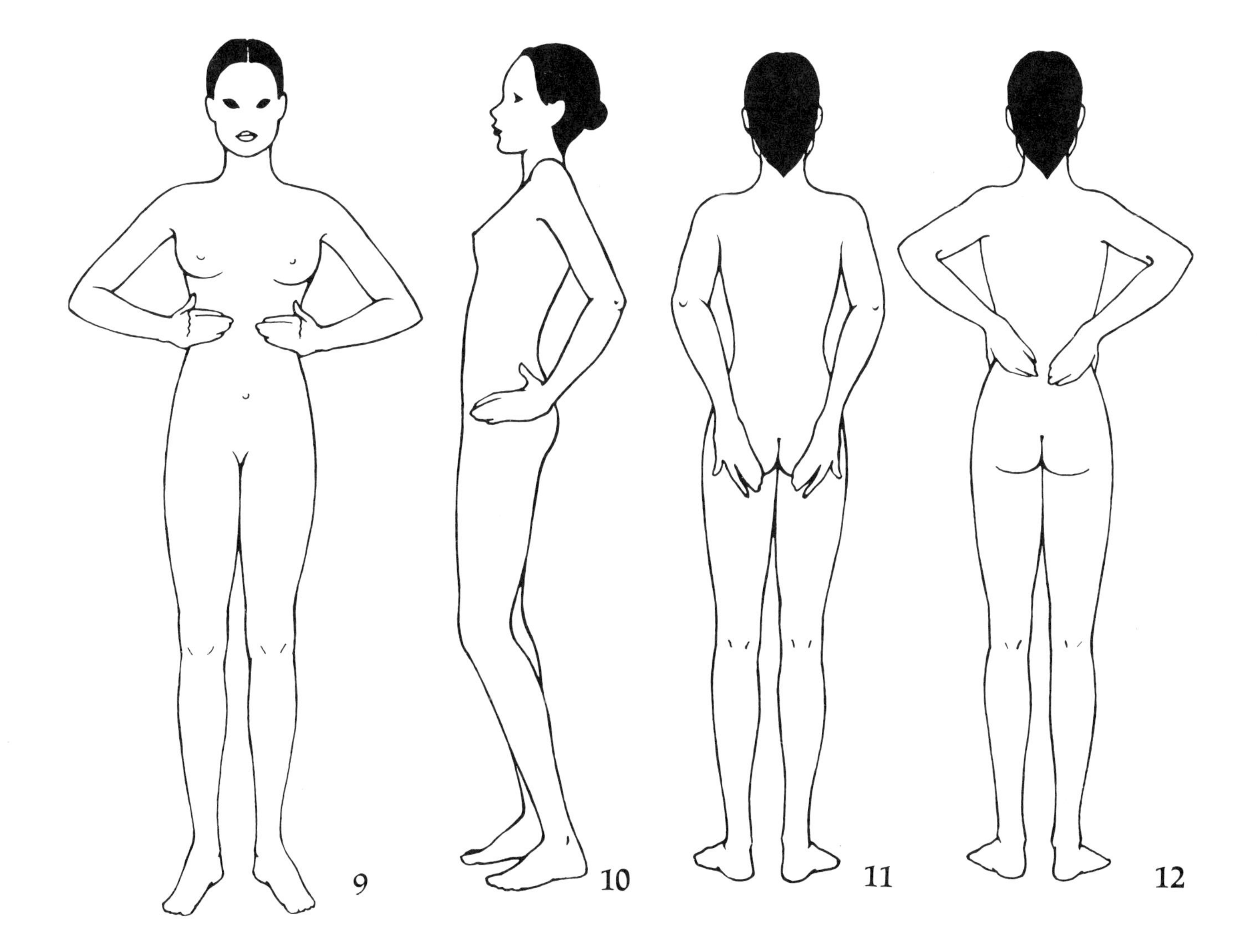

THE NECK

RELAXER

Here, where it is difficult to stay looking young and unlined, play the water on to the neck and start in position **13** with the fingers of the hand and the pads of the fingers pressing against the neck, not too hard, on either side of the voice-box and draw them up as shown in **14** to the margin of the chin, and then start all over again. Do this at least ten times.

After a day's work there are many aches and pains at the base of the neck and you can help loosen up the muscles there, besides getting a good line, by taking position **15**.

SOOTHER

Press hard with the fingertips and draw them up in a smooth sweeping motion, with the water playing on your neck, into position **16**. Do this at least ten times.

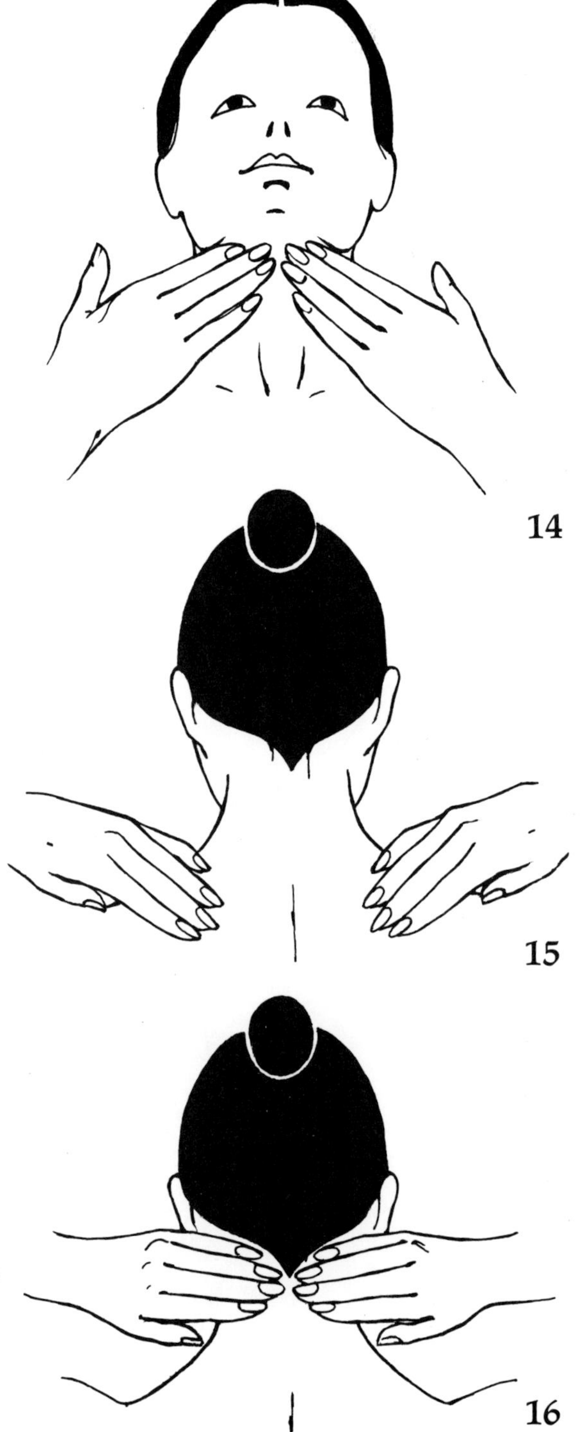

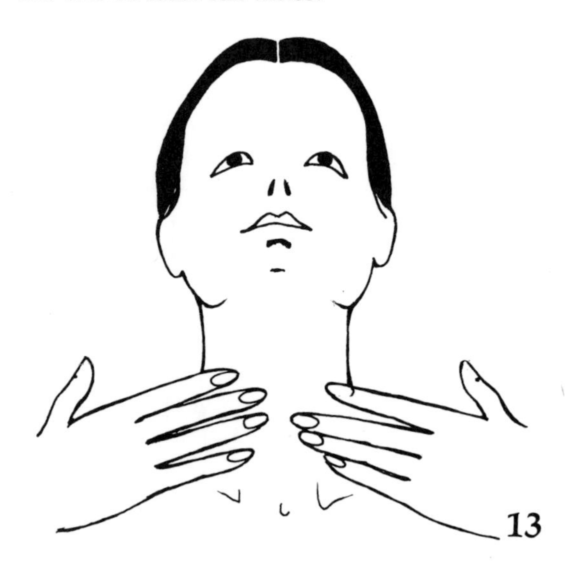

THE LEGS

The legs are often neglected and this leads to varicose veins too early in life, but you can guard against this by doing the following massage schedule.

BODY CONTOURER

Starting at **17**, press on each side of the leg with palms and fingers of each hand drawing them up until you get to the knee. Pressing hard all the time, continue with the hand on the inside of the thigh going right up to the crotch, as shown in **18**, with the other hand now on the hip. Repeat this at least five times for each leg.

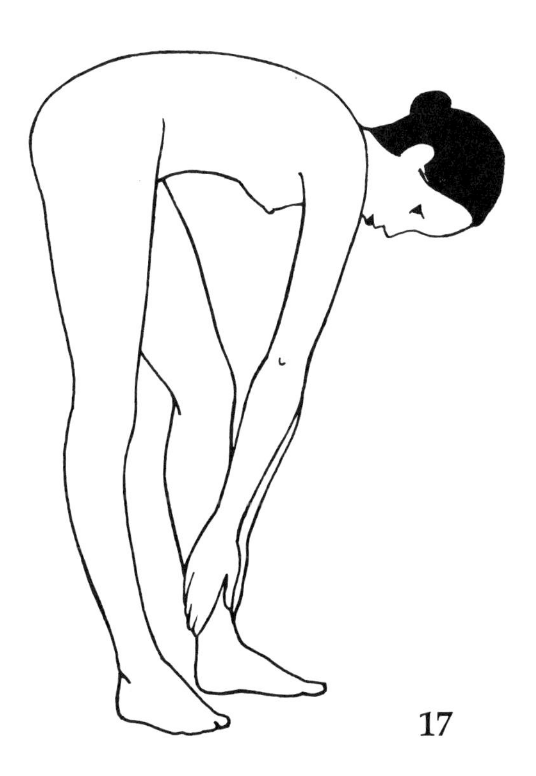

17

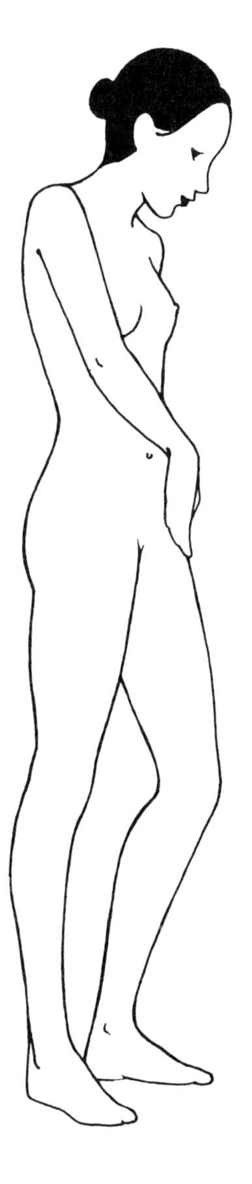

18

THE BUTTOCKS

With one hand, as shown in drawing **19**, draw it up, pressing hard on to the middle of the back, **20**, and then swoop round as shown in **21**, on to your breast. When you get strong enough, this can be done with both hands at the same time. It is always a good idea to work very hard on the waist, drawing up from the buttocks.

THE BREASTS

You can also work on your breasts as shown in **22**, pressing up from underneath them with both hands, up over them as the water cascades down and then up to the neck, to produce a good line from neck to breast as shown in **23**.

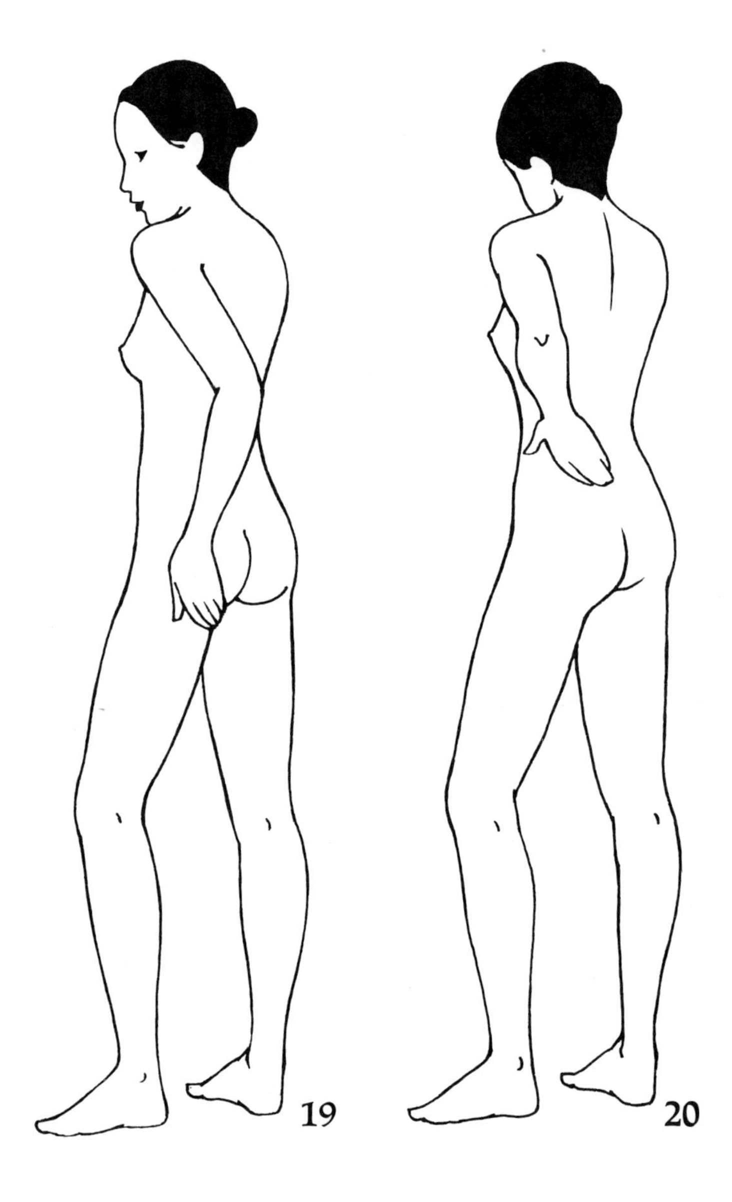

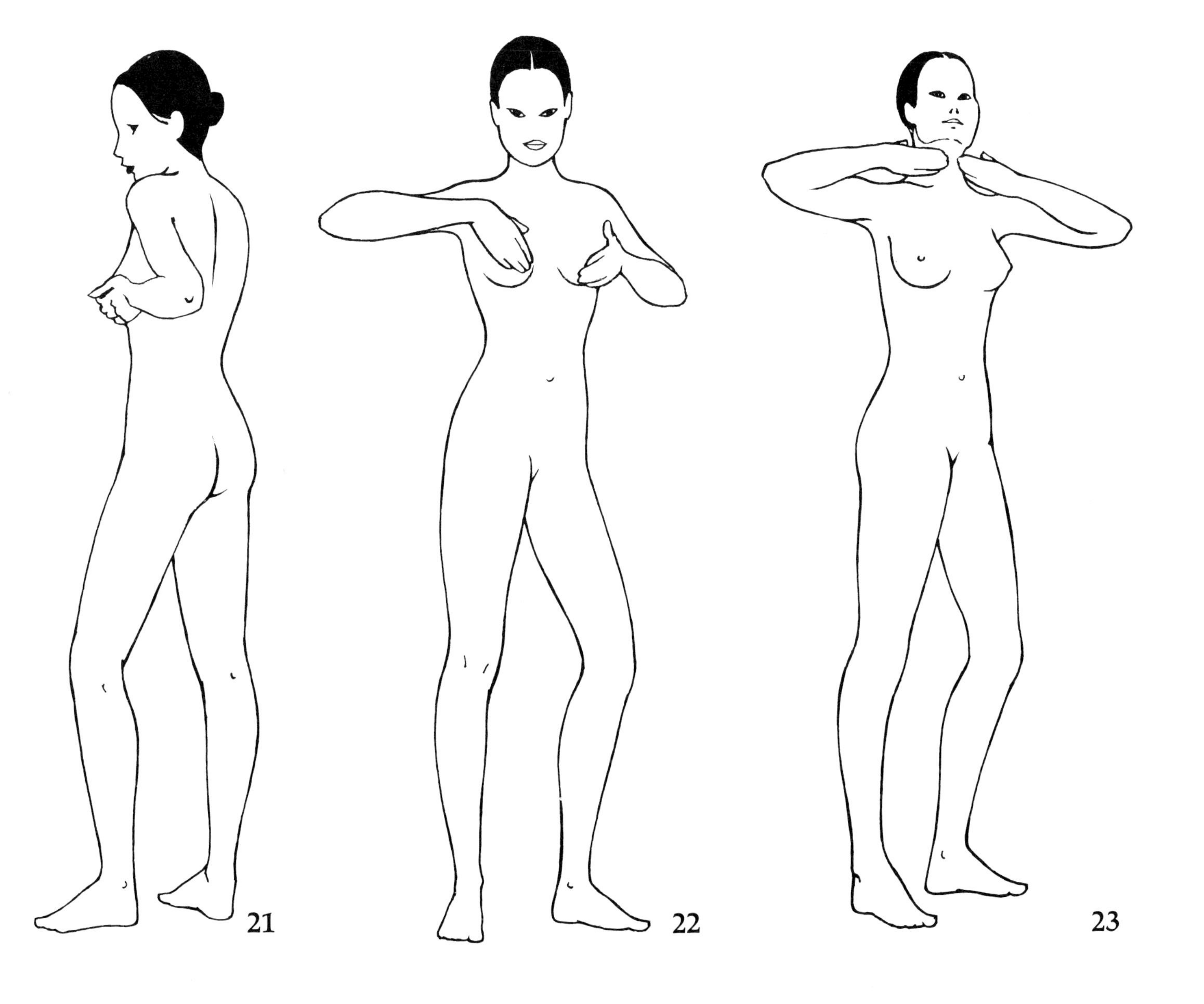
21
22
23

Massage in the Bath

Massage in the bath has the advantage that you can sit down while you are doing it and have the parts of the body you are massaging totally immersed in water.

THE LEGS

THE SLIDE

Good work can be done on making the blood flow and removing soreness and cramps in the muscles as shown in **24** where the fingertips are pushed deeply into the back of the leg and are then pulled up towards the back of the thigh. In **25** you can see how the inside of the top of the thigh can be massaged in one continuous motion.

This position for the massage can also be used for underneath the leg.

24

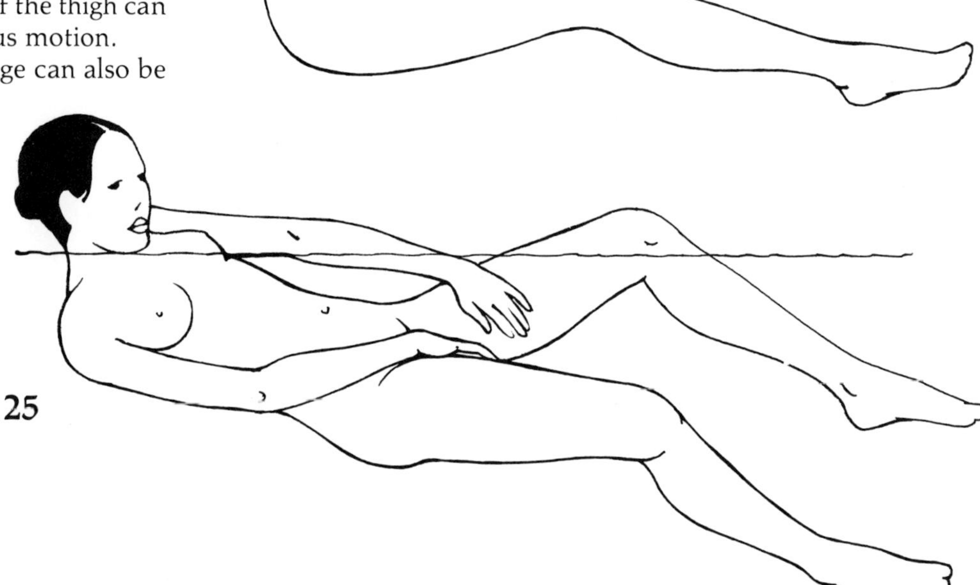

25

ANTI-CELLULITE MASSAGE

Removal of cellulite from the buttocks can be aided by a sequence shown in **26** and **27** where the work on the top of the buttocks is to be seen, and in **28** for work on the inside of the thigh with both hands. This motion on the inside of the thigh can be taken over with both hands on each side of the crotch as shown in **29** and continued right up as in **30** to the tummy, thereby getting a good line in this area where flab accumulates. Some work for the waist is to be found in **31** where the positions of the hands and the power used in the hands are rather similar to those used under the shower. In **32** there is some work that can be done on the bust, but generally speaking it is far better to do this under a shower.

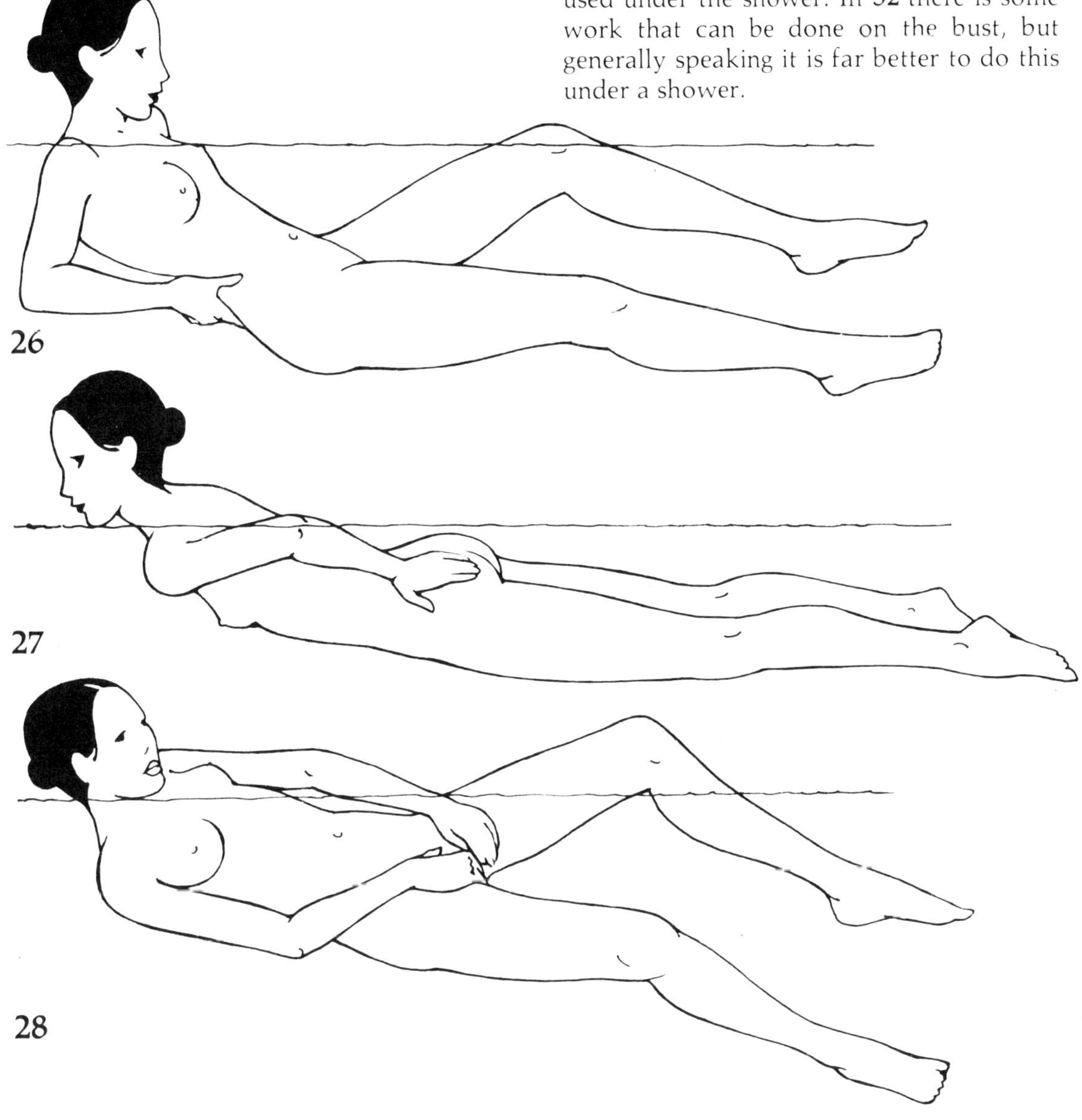

26

27

28

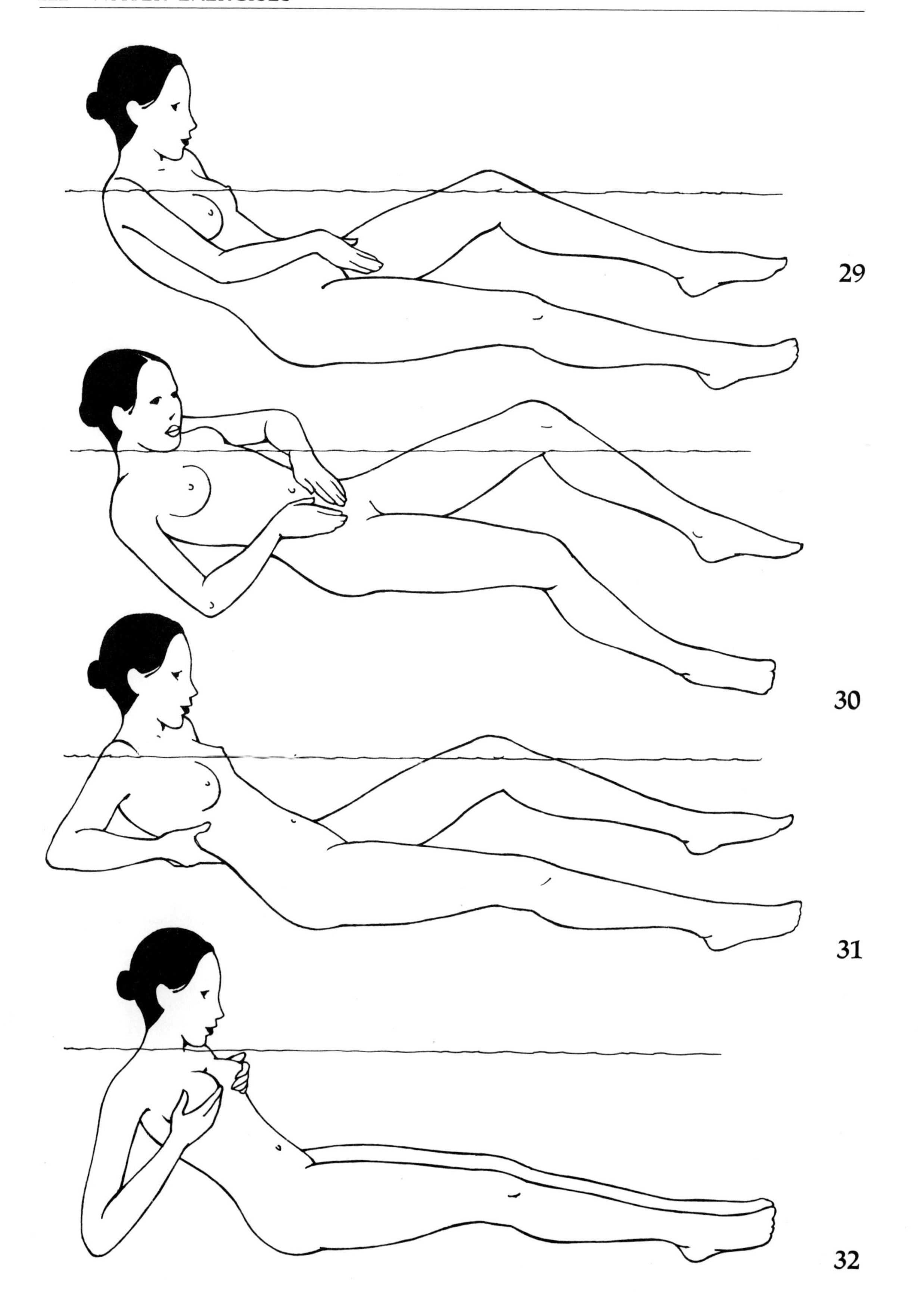
29
30
31
32

Using your Towel as a Masseur

This sequence shows you how, when you are drying yourself on the beach or after a swim, shower or bath, you can use the towel with the invigorating and figure-forming effects of massage. Here the effect is rather different from using the shower as an aid to massage because this time you are working on invigorating the blood supply rather than smoothing the skin. The towelling also gets rid of dead skin and produces a very good sheen.

THE SHEENER

You can work on the legs beginning with position **33** and drawing up similarly with the shower massage to the top of the thigh; then you can work on the front and back of the legs as shown in **34**. By continuing the movement you can come on to the waist and tummy, pressing hard all the time. Very powerful effects on the muscle tone of the upper thigh can be achieved by taking position **35**, and the buttocks can be invigorated by using **36**, and the waist in **37**. In all cases, pull quite hard, but not hard enough to burn the skin, using a backward and forward motion of the towel. Additional work can be done on the tummy by pressing hard and going in a circular movement around each side of the navel, as shown in **38**.

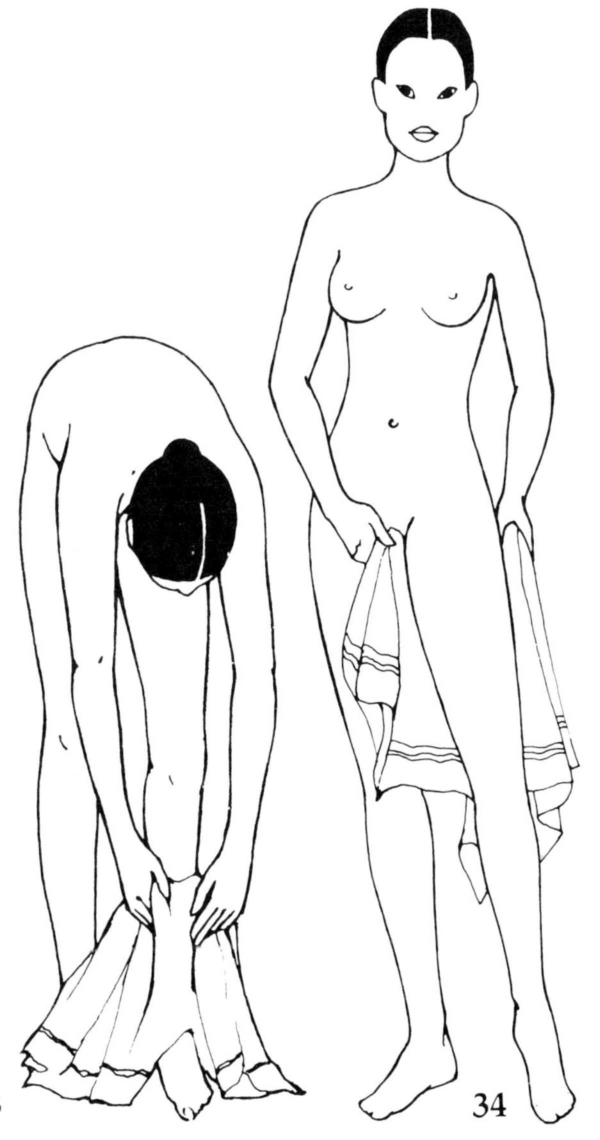

33 34

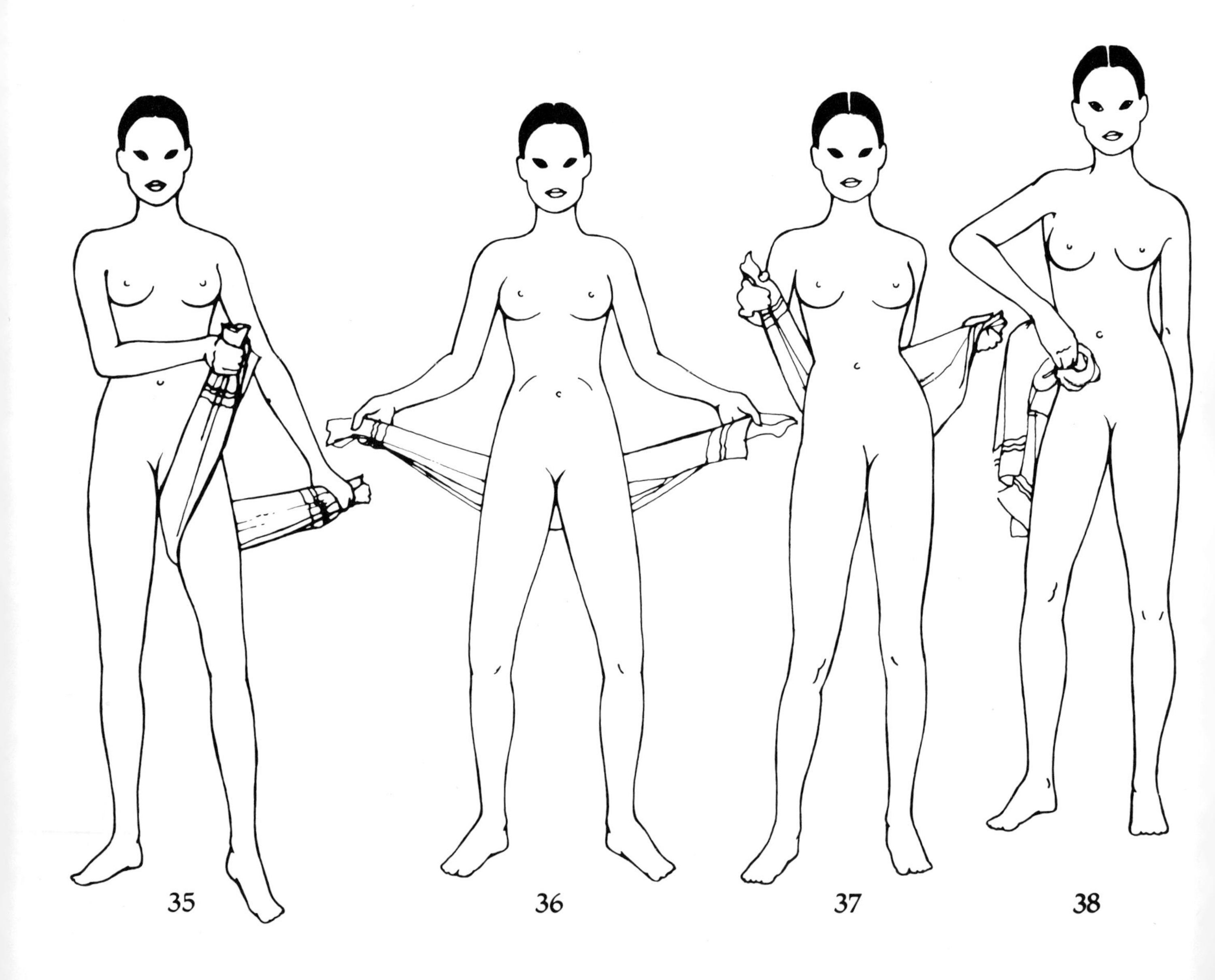
35
36
37
38

Chapter Ten

ADVANCED WATER MASSAGE

ADVANCED WATER MASSAGE

When you are floating in water, either on your back or by taking a deep breath and lying flat these massage techniques can be used very well, because it is as if you were floating on a perfect bed. Other people can also massage you.

ATHENE

In **1**, where you would be in water up to the knee, you can see how the backs of the legs can be massaged. Press hard and use the fingertips from the Achilles tendon up to the back of the knee, stroking upwards and then repeating by starting at the bottom and working up again. It is very good for legs that get tired from too much standing on feet all day.

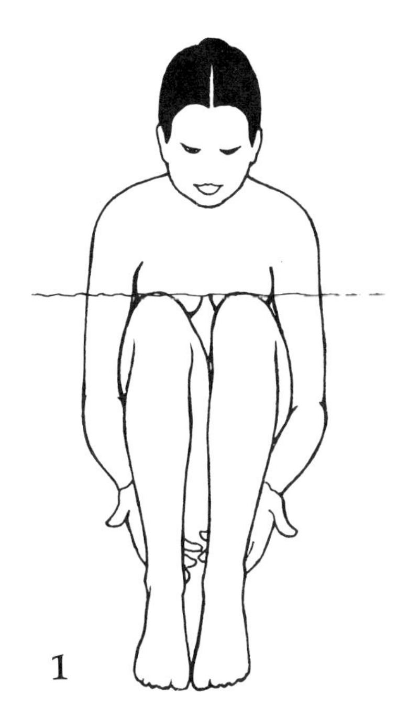

1

DIANA

In **2** you see how you can use your fingertips below the knee to press, which helps remove tension in the leg, and also improves the health of the joint. Here you press, hold for a couple of seconds, then relax. Press again. This can be done in water just covering the knee.

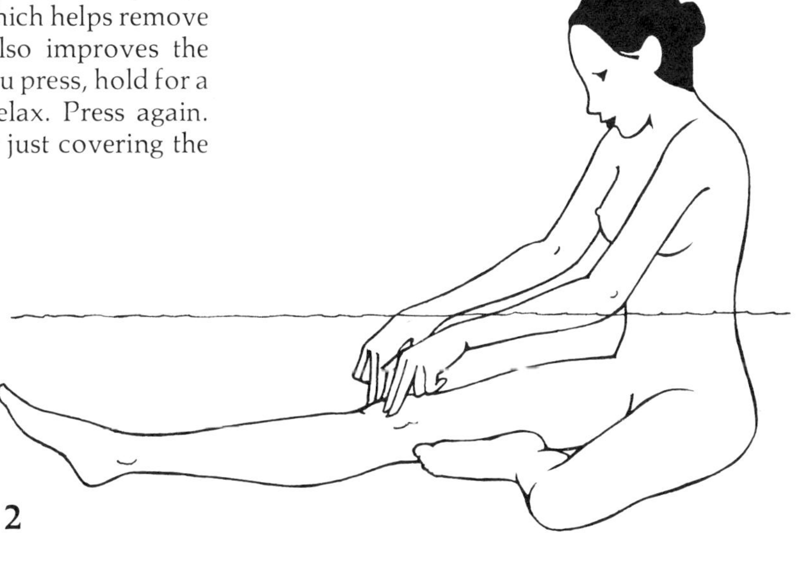

2

THE REJUVENATOR

In sequence, **3, 4** and **5,** you can see how the fingertips are used on the inside of the leg, coming up over the calf. Note particularly the position of the fingers in **4,** where they are at the top of the knee and pressing on the thick tendons of the knee joint. Move up into the top of the thigh. Press quite hard here on the way up. This will exercise your fingers.

Next, in **6**, there is the use of three fingers pressing deeply on either side of the navel and on the strong muscles that go down from the chest to the pubic arch. You find them by coughing, pressing your fingers, and moving across from the centre of the tummy until you reach the position shown in **6**, when you have come to the edge of the muscles. Don't press too hard. Just press and relax, then press again. The useful thing is to have water covering that area of the body. In **7** you can see where a very powerful press on the buttocks along with the work in **6** is a very good toner of this part of the body. It is used often to effect over-all weight loss and slimming.

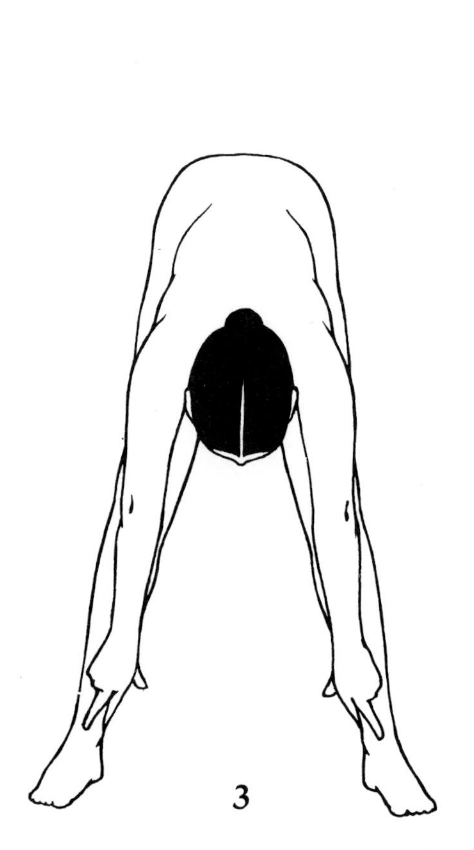

3

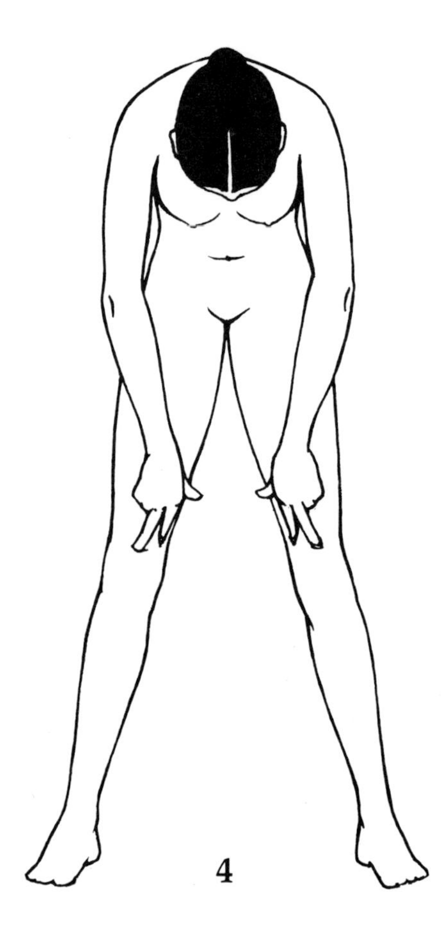

4

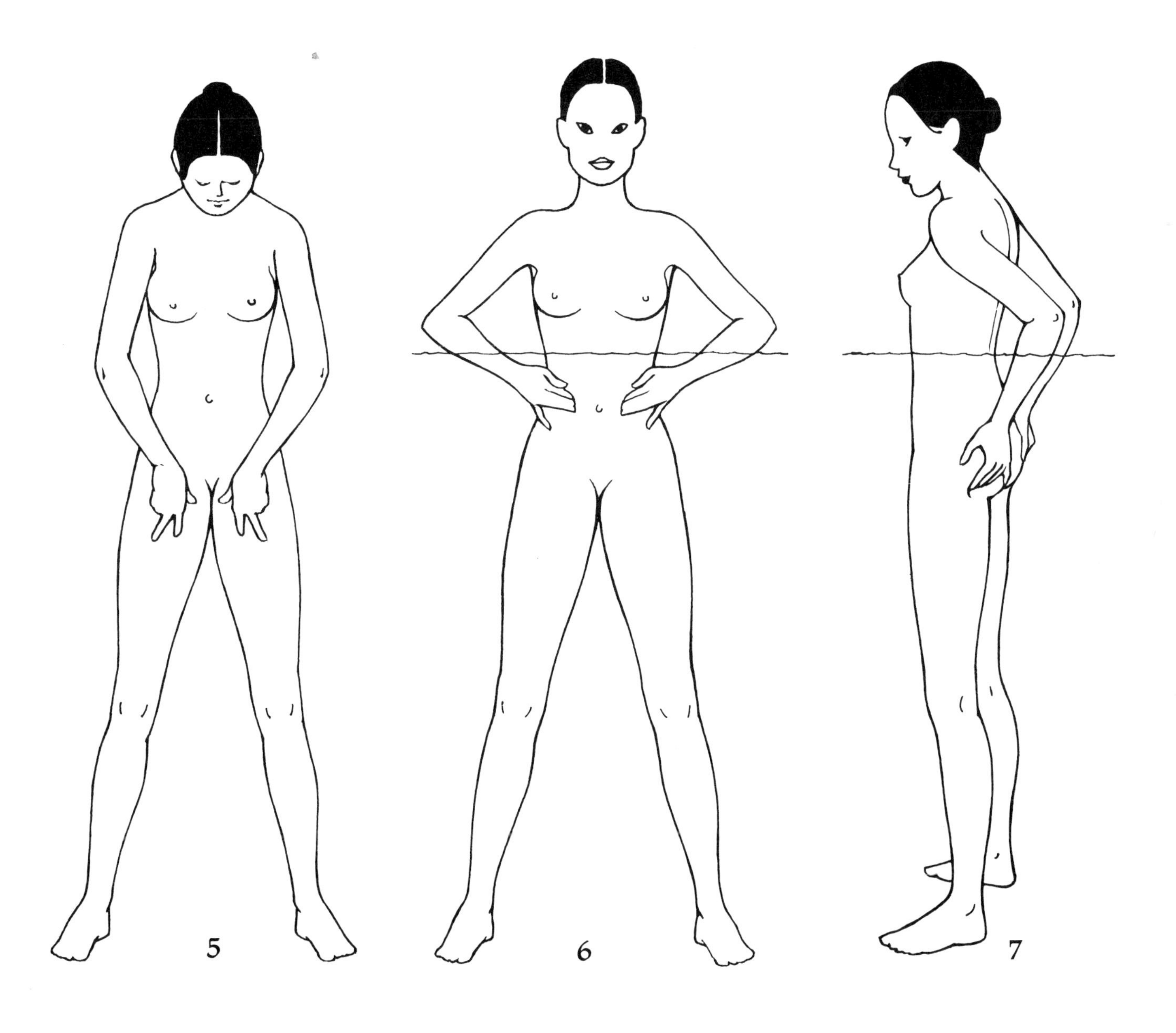
5
6
7

FRONT VENUS LINES

More extended work on the front of the tummy and the breasts is shown in **8.** The lower area marked 'A', is to be massaged by pressing the fingers deeply into the flesh—not to cause pain, of course—circling by moving the hand in a rotary motion, and then after a few seconds stopping, then beginning again. A similar method is used for 'B'. Both these exercises reduce the tension in the pelvic floor, and tone the body generally. The pathway shown by the arrowed line in 'C' means that you begin on one side and with your finger-tips work round just underneath the rib-cage and down again. Do this several times in one direction, then repeat in another direction. You will find this is very relaxing indeed. 'D' has the same effect, but you are working on the breasts this time. This is a very good exercise (as is 'C') underneath the shower. Bring your fingertips down from one side, following the line of the arrow in this quite complicated but pretty shape. Start again several times, and then switch direction.

All these movements, from 'A' to 'D', can be done on yourself in the shower, or they can also be done by somebody else for you when you are lying on your back, floating, in the water. It is best done in warmish water than cold. The result is particularly soothing and pleasant.

In 9 the areas 'E', 'F' and 'G' are to be quite strongly massaged with the fingertips together, or the palm of the hand, or the heel of the hand. If you are lying in water and somebody stands between your legs, they can press the heel of the hand along 'E' from the pubic arch up; for 'F', underneath the breast and down into the armpit; for 'G', on the inside of the breast in a curving motion up. In all cases you move upwards from the

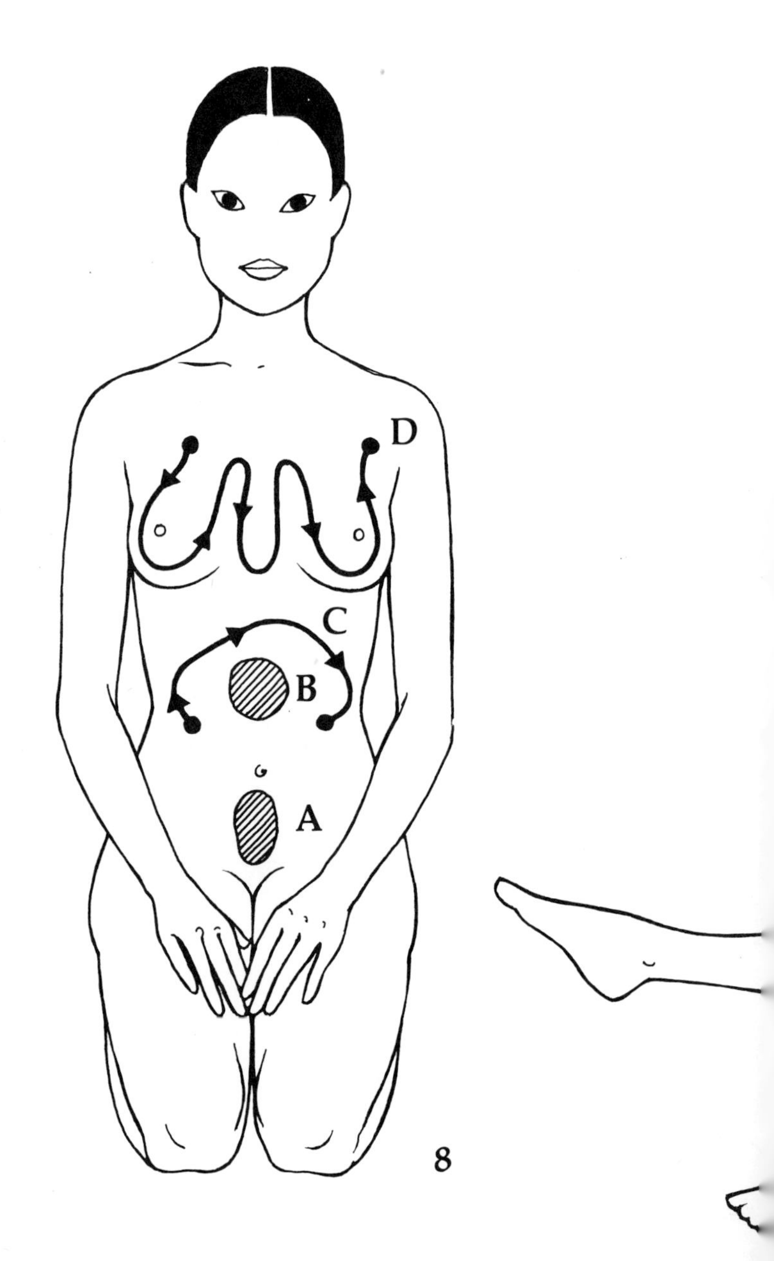

8

feet. Up, then down again, then up. Press quite hard going up, take your time doing it and come down very gently. The water provides very good lubrication for this.

BACK VENUS LINES

In **10** you get very good shaping of the body and vitalisation by the lines 'H' and 'I'. You start in 'H' from the lower point and move up in a wide curving line to end up on the opposite buttock. With 'I' you start more centrally in the back of the knee, work up on the outside of the buttock and end up at the waist. In these movements, starting in the direction shown, always work *up*, not down. This exercise is best done in the water, in which case your partner will have to stand behind and work upwards, if you are standing; but if you are lying in the starfish position, lying face downwards, someone standing between your legs can do this. When they get very expert, you can lie on your back and they can stand beside you and follow up that line. The drawings show 'H' on the left leg and 'I' on the right leg, but of course you do *both* of these lines on *both* legs.

9

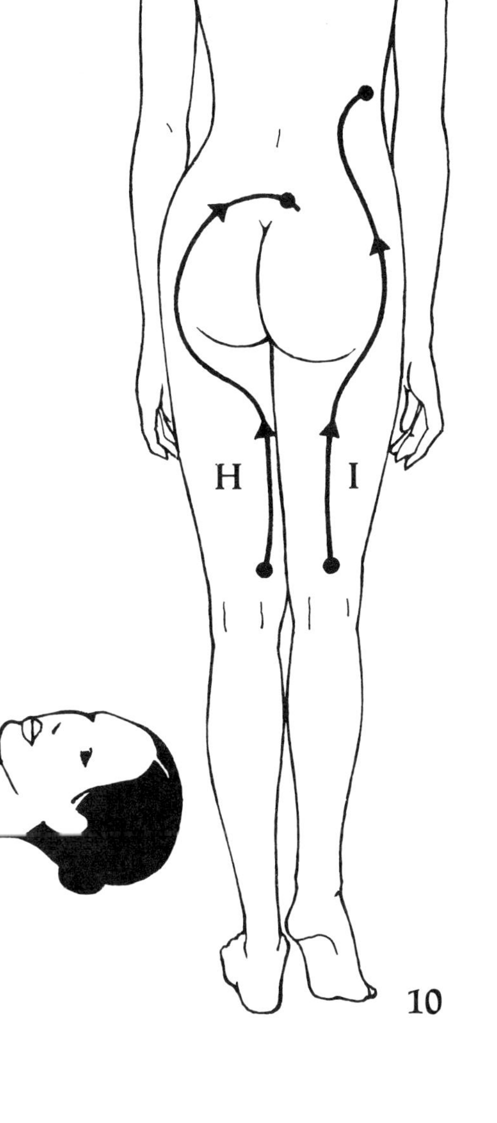

10

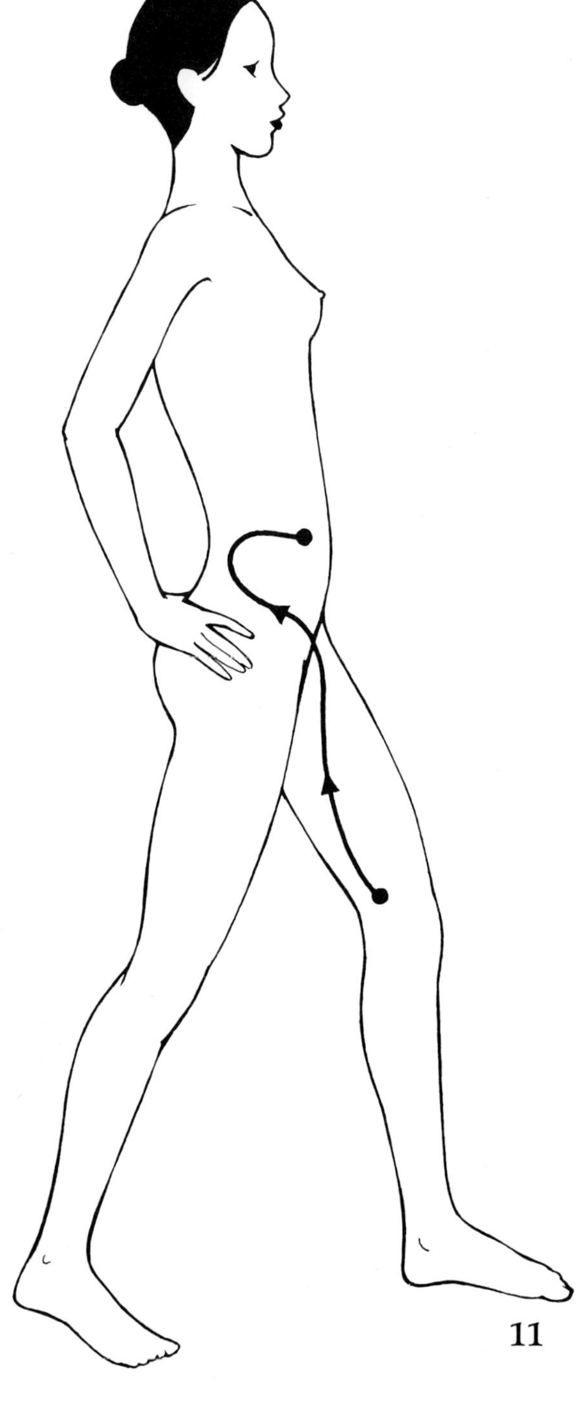

11

SIDE VENUS LINES

In **11** you see a very advanced line on the inside of the leg, following up to the top of the thigh, crossing over the crotch, across the hip into a curve in the back and then to the tummy. Again this can be done in the shower or it can be done when you are lying flat on your back in the water or when you are standing in water. The drawing shows the line beginning on the left leg. You do both legs, of course.

SUPER VENUS LINES

In **12** you have some very good lines. The technique is as previously described—you could be standing in your shower, or lying on your back in the water with someone else doing the work, standing between your legs or to one side. Remember that the work is from the lower body up to the higher part.

When first trying these massage techniques it is best to take the most simple position. It is a good idea to learn to do them on dry land using a sun cream or a moisturising cream on the body. As you and your friends get more expert, you can move to the shower, and eventually you'll be able to use the very best technique, which is done lying in the water. After a while you can vary the positions; not of the lines but of the position of the body when it is being massaged. In chapter 9 there are at least a dozen excellent positions to take.

This is a *doing* book and if you *do* do the exercises in the previous chapters and the massage techniques that follow, and eventually combine them, you will have no doubt at all about their efficacy for reducing tension, bringing relaxation, creating pleasure inside your body, getting to know other people well and getting to know yourself well. They will improve the vitality and general tone of your body, cast off aches and pains after a tiring working day, loosen your joints and help you towards an exhilarating sense of fitness and well-being.

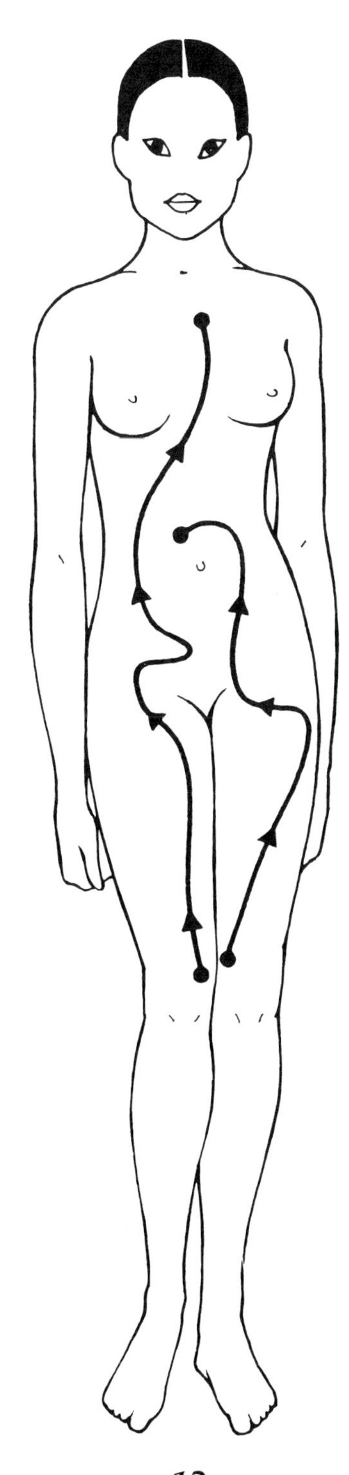

12